2018

Annual Health Reform Update

Sara E. Wilensky, JD, PhD
The George Washington University
Milken Institute School of Public Health
Department of Health Policy and Management
Washington, DC

Joel B. Teitelbaum, JD, LLM
The George Washington University
Milken Institute School of Public Health
Department of Health Policy and Management
Washington, DC

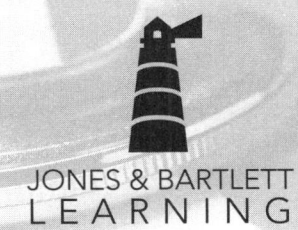

JONES & BARTLETT
LEARNING

World Headquarters
Jones & Bartlett Learning
5 Wall Street
Burlington, MA 01803
978-443-5000
info@jblearning.com
www.jblearning.com

Jones & Bartlett Learning books and products are available through most bookstores and online booksellers. To contact Jones & Bartlett Learning directly, call 800-832-0034, fax 978-443-8000, or visit our website, www.jblearning.com.

> Substantial discounts on bulk quantities of Jones & Bartlett Learning publications are available to corporations, professional associations, and other qualified organizations. For details and specific discount information, contact the special sales department at Jones & Bartlett Learning via the above contact information or send an email to specialsales@jblearning.com.

Production Credits

VP, Executive Publisher: David D. Cella
Publisher: Michael Brown
Associate Editor: Danielle Bessette
Associate Production Editor: Alex Schab
Senior Marketing Manager: Sophie Fleck Teague
Production Services Manager: Colleen Lamy
Manufacturing and Inventory Control Supervisor: Amy Bacus
Composition: SourceHOV LLC

Cover Design: Kristin E. Parker
Director of Rights & Media: Joanna Gallant
Rights & Media Specialist: Merideth Tumasz
Media Development Editor: Shannon Sheehan
Cover Image (Title Page, Chapter Opener): © Andy Dean Photography/ShutterStock, Inc.
Printing and Binding: Edwards Brothers Malloy
Cover Printing: Edwards Brothers Malloy

ISBN: 978-1-284-15034-6

6048

Printed in the United States of America
21 20 19 18 17   10 9 8 7 6 5 4 3 2 1

2018 Annual Health Reform Update

LEARNING OBJECTIVES

By the end of this text you will be able to:

- Describe previous national health reform attempts
- Understand why national health reform has been difficult to achieve in the United States
- Analyze why national health reform succeeded in 2010 when so many previous attempts had failed
- Understand the key components of the Patient Protection and Affordable Care Act
- Understand the core rulings of multiple U.S. Supreme Court decisions related to the Affordable Care Act
- Evaluate the political climate regarding repealing and replacing the Affordable Care Act, and understand the main features of legislation drafted toward that end
- Describe key issues going forward related to implementation of the Affordable Care Act

▶ Introduction

The Patient Protection and Affordable Care Act (generally referred to as the Affordable Care Act, or ACA) is the most monumental piece of U.S. federal health policymaking in nearly 50 years. It reorders not only many aspects of the health insurance and healthcare delivery systems but also long-standing relationships that underpin those systems. Yet beyond the sheer scope and content of the ACA and the policy trade-offs that led to its passage lies another story: its implementation and subsequent effect on the lives of tens of millions of Americans. Implementation of the ACA is an ongoing, dynamic process for the federal government, states, employers, insurers, providers, patients, and others. In addition, there have been and, no doubt, will continue to be state and federal court decisions across the country that alter the trajectory of the law and its implementation.

VIGNETTE

A group of friends were talking about the Affordable Care Act (ACA), illustrating the wide-ranging viewpoints about the law. Calvin, whose daughter Mia is struggling to make a living as an artist, is pleased that Mia has health insurance for the first time since graduating from college. Although Mia cannot stay on her parents' insurance because she just turned 27, she can now afford a good health insurance plan that she found on her state's health exchange. While Calvin has not noticed much of a change in his own health insurance coverage, which he obtains through his government employer, his friend Katherine is upset about health reform. She does not want the government forcing her to purchase health insurance (although she always chose to be insured in the past), and she recently found out that her old plan was cancelled because it did not meet the law's requirements. Katherine found several new plan options to choose from, but none had her exact combination of benefits, providers, and price. In addition, Katherine's uncle, Ethan, is 55 years old and self-employed. He purchases his health insurance on his state's exchange and because he has preexisting conditions, he is grateful to be able to find a plan. Even so, Ethan's premiums will increase by 15% this year and his deductible is $5,000, making health care difficult to afford even with insurance. Another friend, Jara, told Katherine she should be willing to pay a little more or change some aspects of her plan to help the millions of people who can now afford insurance for the first time as a result of the ACA. After witnessing her uncle's experience, however, Katherine is skeptical that the government is going to be able to keep its promises.

This vignette fairly describes just a few of the competing viewpoints about the ACA and its role in creating a new and potentially more equitable health insurance system. As ACA implementation moves forward, bear in mind the many different ways that this round of health reform can be perceived and how it affects people differently.

Furthermore, the future of the ACA was made even more uncertain by the monumental election cycle in 2016. Unexpectedly, Donald Trump was elected president in November of that year, and the Republicans maintained control of both the U.S. House of Representatives and the Senate. Having control of Congress and the White House gives Republicans a chance to fulfill a promise they have campaigned on for years—to repeal and replace the ACA. Even if they are not successful in passing a repeal and replacement bill, President Trump can use his executive powers to rewrite existing regulations and implement new policies. Indeed, he has already started to do so, as will be discussed later.

The interplay between legal and political decisions makes it difficult to discern how implementation of the law will be carried out, assuming it is not repealed entirely. By way of example, the U.S. Supreme Court's landmark 2012 decision upholding the constitutionality of the ACA and 2015 decision upholding subsidies provided through the ACA to the federal insurance exchange are described in the pages that follow, and there are currently dozens of lawsuits challenging the ACA's coverage mandate related to contraceptive and other family planning services. The practical consequences and legal rulings that actually manifest as a result of ACA implementation—not just the changes to American health care contemplated by Congress when they put pen to paper with the ACA—will, for years to come, need to be studied and understood by students across a range of disciplines, not just for academic purposes, but for healthcare and public health job market purposes as well.

Although there has been general agreement about the problems facing the U.S. healthcare system—high costs, high uninsured rates, health disparities, quality concerns—politicians and voters have disagreed about the best solutions. As a result, numerous attempts to pass national health reform legislation did not succeed. What was different in 2010? Why was the Obama administration successful when several previous attempts had failed? This text begins with a discussion of why it has been so difficult to achieve broad health reform in this country, and then examines the numerous failed attempts at national health reform over the last century. It then analyzes how health reform was enacted in 2010, provides an overview of the law that eventually emerged, and covers the U.S. Supreme Court decision upholding its constitutionality. Finally, this text moves to a discussion of the current political climate and what it means for health reform going forward, including a discussion of key political and implementation issues. Throughout this text we examine several key themes: choosing between state flexibility and national uniformity; determining the appropriate role for government, the private sector, and the healthcare financing and delivery entities; defining a primary decision-making goal (e.g., fiscal restraint, equity/social justice, improved health outcomes, uniformity); and settling on the appropriate scope of coverage to offer beneficiaries.

▶ Difficulty Achieving Health Reform in the United States

The array of problems facing the healthcare system has led to numerous health reform proposals and implemented policies. The concept of health reform can have several different meanings. Given the patchwork health insurance system, health reform often refers to changes that seek to reduce the number of uninsured. Due to the high and increasing cost of healthcare services, health reform might also include changes that seek to contain costs and control utilization. The notion of health reform could also address other shortcomings, such as trying to reduce medical errors, strengthening patient rights, building the public health infrastructure, and confronting the rising cost of medical malpractice insurance. Unsurprisingly, the ACA, the federal health reform law passed in 2010, touches on many of these issues.[1]

We begin with a discussion about why health reform is difficult to achieve in the United States and then introduce some of the reforms that have been attempted, with varying degrees of success, on a national level. Numerous authors have addressed the main factors that deter significant social reform in this country, including health reform.[2-4] Factors that are prominently discussed include the country's culture, the nature of U.S. political institutions, the power of interest groups, and path dependency (i.e., the notion that people are generally opposed to change).

Culture

This country's culture and lack of consensus about health reform have impeded attempts to create universal coverage health plans. The twin concepts of entrepreneurialism and individualism have had a real impact on health policy decisions: Americans generally oppose government solutions to social welfare problems.[4(p438)]

In addition, there is no agreement about the overall scope of the healthcare problems we face.[5] Prior to the passage of the ACA, most Americans believed the extant health system needed major changes, yet 22% believed only minor changes were required and another 17% thought the system should basically stay the same.[5]

Americans have a complicated and partisan view of the proper role of the federal government in the healthcare arena. On one hand, 60% of respondents to a 2017 survey felt that the federal government has a responsibility to ensure healthcare coverage for all Americans.[7] This is much higher than the 47% who shared that view in 2010, at the height of the health reform debate.[8] Of those who supported federal intervention in the 2017 survey, 33% would like to see a single-payer system developed.[7]

At the same time, there was a stark difference of opinion based on the respondent's political views. While 85% of Democrats and Democrat-leaning independents believed the federal government was responsible for ensuring healthcare coverage, only 32% of Republicans and Republican-leaning independents agreed.[7] Even so, over half (57%) of Republican/Republican-leaners supported the continuation of Medicaid and Medicare, the country's largest public health insurance programs. Furthermore, only 5% of respondents thought the federal government should not have any role in ensuring healthcare coverage.[7]

It is accepted political dogma that it is difficult to take away benefits once they are established, and this has proven to be true with healthcare coverage.[9] The popularity of the ACA has increased since the Republicans gained power in the 2016 elections and the threat of repealing the ACA became a realistic possibility. A June 2017 Kaiser Tracking poll showed the ACA's favorability ratings above 50% for the first time since the poll began in 2010,[10] and a separate poll taken a couple months later showed 64% of respondents preferred to either keep the ACA as it is or make fixes to it that would shore up problems and weaknesses.[11] Furthermore, the public is clearly opposed to the proposed Republican replacement plans. A majority of respondents opposed both the House (56% opposed)[12] and Senate (55% opposed)[13] bills. Even though many Republicans also opposed the replacement options (only 21% have a very favorable view),[10] most Republicans (about 75%) would still like to see the ACA repealed and replaced at some point.[11]

U.S. Political System

The country's system of government also has made it difficult to achieve universal coverage. Traditionally, social welfare programs—including the provision of health care—have been the responsibility of the states. Initially, there was almost no federal involvement in the provision of health care, and when the federal government became more heavily involved in 1965, Medicaid continued to keep the locus of decision making at the state level. Of course, there are select populations, such as the elderly (Medicare) and veterans (Veterans Health Administration), who have a federalized health insurance system. However, the country appears to support a Medicaid-type expansion over a new federalized program.[8]

Although states are generally home to social welfare changes, it is difficult to provide universal health care on a state-by-state basis. If state health reform efforts lead the way, the country could have a patchwork of programs and policies that vary from state to state, with the potential to make health coverage even more complex and inefficient than it is currently. In addition, states must consider whether they are making policy decisions that will give employers an incentive to choose to locate in another state with fewer or less onerous legal requirements. If employers leave the state, it could result in loss of jobs and have downstream effects on the state's economy.

The federal government also has resource advantages over states, making it easier for the federal level to be the engine for health reform. Individual states have a much smaller tax and revenue base than the federal government to draw from to implement health reform plans. In addition, once the federal government decides to tax a good or service, a state's ability to tax that same good or service is constrained by the individual's willingness and ability to pay a higher price. Unlike the federal government, most states have some type of balanced budget requirement.[14] While state legislatures may use accounting gimmicks and other maneuvers to avoid balanced budget requirements, states more often must make difficult choices about resource allocation that federal policymakers often avoid (and thus generate enormous deficits). These restrictions, however, also may help with reform efforts by forcing states to a crisis point where a decision must be made to avoid an untenable situation. The federal government rarely reaches such a crisis point, which means tough decisions are often left for the next Congress, executive branch administration, or generation.

State reform efforts are also constrained by the Employee Retirement Income Security Act of 1974 (ERISA). ERISA is a federal law that regulates "welfare benefit programs," including health plans, operated by private employers. ERISA limits ability of states to reform because it broadly preempts state laws that "relate to" employer-sponsored plans and because it applies to nearly all individuals who receive health benefits through a private employer. One effect of the law, for example, is that states have little regulatory control over the benefits covered in employer-sponsored health plans, because ERISA accords employers near-total discretion over the design of their benefit packages.[15(p237)]

Despite these hurdles, it is also important to recognize that a health reform strategy focusing on states has benefits as well. At its best, state-level reform can be accomplished more rapidly and with more innovation than at the federal level. State legislatures may have an easier time convincing a narrower band of constituents important to the state than Congress has in accommodating the varied needs of stakeholders nationwide. Along the same lines, states are able to target reforms to meet the particular needs of their population, instead of covering more diverse needs across the entire country. Additionally, through the use of "direct democracy" (referenda, ballot initiatives, etc.), it is easier for citizens to have an impact on decisions by state-level policymakers than by federal legislators. Finally, because the healthcare delivery system is run primarily on the state level, states have the expertise and ability to implement many parts of healthcare reform.

Other aspects of the U.S. political system also make it difficult to institute sweeping reform. For example, although presidents have significant influence on policy agenda-setting and proposing budgets, they have limited power to make changes without the assistance of Congress. The federal government is often politically divided, with different parties holding power in the executive and legislative branches. This division often results in partisanship and policy inaction due to different policy priorities and views.

Furthermore, although members of Congress may ride the coattails of a popular president from their own party, they are not reliant on the president to keep their jobs. The issues and views their constituents care about most may not align with the president's priorities. In those cases, members of Congress have a strong incentive to adhere to the wishes of those who vote for them, instead of simply following the president's lead. Barring an overwhelming wave of discontent, as occurred in the 2010 midterm elections when Democrats suffered historic losses in Congress, it is usually difficult to unseat incumbents. Even when there is a historic level of turnover, reelection rates remain very high. For example, 97% of House incumbents successfully defended their seats in 2016; even in the Senate, where turnover is relatively more common, 93% of incumbents won reelection in 2016.[16] As a result, legislators in Congress may have confidence in focusing on their district's or state's needs before those of the entire nation.

Federal legislative rules also support inaction or incremental reform over sweeping changes. In the Senate, 60 (of 100) votes are needed to break a filibuster in most cases. Thus, even the political party in the majority can have difficulty effectuating change. One exception to the filibuster rule is the "reconciliation" process, which allows bills to pass with only 51 votes. Reconciliation is used as part of the budgetary process and bills passed via reconciliation may not be filibustered (so can pass with 51 votes), can only pertain to federal revenue and spending issues, must comply with spending and revenue targets set forth in the budget resolution, and must adhere to other budgetary rules.[17] The reconciliation process is being increasingly used when one party maintains a slim majority and that party cannot find 60 votes to pass a bill. For example, the Democrats used a reconciliation bill to pass the ACA in 2010 after they lost their filibuster-proof majority, and likewise, the Republicans attempted to use a reconciliation bill to pass their ACA repeal-and-replace bills. Also, because both the House and the Senate have to pass bills containing the same policies and language to have any chance at becoming law, a large political majority in one chamber or the other does not guarantee the ability to enact a policy. As a result, in many cases members of Congress have to work together, at least to some degree, to devise a consensus policy that satisfies enough members to pass a bill. This need to build consensus makes radical change unlikely.

Interest Groups

Interest groups often influence the decisions of politicians. The role of interest groups is to represent their members' interests in policy decisions. These groups can be corporate for-profit entities or nonprofit consumer-oriented organizations. They lobby politicians and the general public about the virtues or vices of specific proposals, work to improve proposals on the policy agenda, and attempt to defeat proposals they believe are not in the best interest of their group. By contributing to political campaigns or by helping to draw supportive voters out on Election Day, interest groups gain the ear, and often the influence, of politicians who vote on issues that are important to the group.

In terms of health reform, interest groups representing various providers, businesses, employer groups, insurance companies, and managed care organizations often have been opposed to comprehensive health reform.[4(pp438-439)] There are numerous points along the path—from developing a policy idea to voting for or against a bill—when interest groups can attempt to affect politicians' views. The more radical the policy proposal, the more interest groups are likely to become engaged in the political decision-making process, making it difficult to pass a bill that includes comprehensive reform.

In general, it is easier to oppose a proposal than to develop one and pass a bill. Opponents of proposals are not required to provide a better alternative to whatever is on the table. Instead, they can simply point to aspects of the policy idea that are unpopular and call for the proposal to be rejected. This was the tactic used by the Health Insurance Association of America in their well-known "Harry and Louise" television ads that opposed the Clinton administration's comprehensive health reform bill in 1993, the Health Security Act. In the ad, Harry and Louise, two "average" Americans, are seen discussing the healthcare system over breakfast. Although they both agree the system needs to be improved, they highlight certain aspects of the Clinton plan that were particularly controversial, such as an overall cap on funds for healthcare needs and restrictions on provider choice. The tag line for the ad was, "There's got to be a better way."[18] Similarly, before the 2016 elections, many Republicans promised to "repeal and replace" the health reform bill without specifying their favored replacement option. To be effective in opposing health reform, opponents did not have to propose an alternative that was scrutinized and compared with the existing proposal. Simply saying "the country can do better" was enough to help create significant opposition to the plan.

Path Dependency

Finally, the concept of path dependency has been a hindrance to major health reform. "The notion of path dependency emphasizes the power of inertia within political institutions."[4(p439)] That is, once a certain way of doing things becomes the norm, it is hard to change course. Yet this theory does not mean that health reform is impossible. Inertia may be overcome at "critical moments or junctures" that open a window for change.[4(p439)] For example, the passage of Medicaid and Medicare in 1965 was a radical change from the past pattern of limited federal government involvement in health care. The catalysts for this change were the growing social pressure for improving the healthcare system and the landslide victory of Democrat Lyndon Johnson as president and of liberal and moderate Democrats in Congress.

The 1992 election of Democrat Bill Clinton, who ran on a platform emphasizing broad health reform, coupled with the Democratic majority in Congress (until 1994), also presented a window of opportunity. Although Clinton's plan was not ultimately successful, it appeared that the American public and politicians were open to changing the course of the healthcare "path" that had been taken to date. In 2010 another "critical moment" appeared, and President Obama took advantage of the circumstances to push through the health reform bill. Although path dependency suggests that inertia and fear of change have made broad reform difficult, it is not impossible to achieve.

Path dependency is also evident on the individual level; that is, once individuals are accustomed to having things a certain way, it is difficult for them to accept change. In 2010, prior to the passage of the ACA, about 84% of Americans had health insurance, most through employer-sponsored coverage.[19] It was assumed that comprehensive health reform would likely change the condition of the insured population to some degree by changing either their source of coverage, the benefits included in coverage, the cost of coverage, or some other factor. During the debate over the ACA, about one-third of people surveyed reported that the bill would probably make them worse off, and another third thought it would not make any difference to them.[5] Professor Judith Feder refers to this problem as the "crowd-out" politics of health reform: "The fundamental barrier to universal coverage is that our success in insuring most of the nation's population has 'crowded out' our political capacity to insure the rest."[20(p461)] In other words, many of the insured do not want a change in the healthcare system that will leave them worse off to make the uninsured better off.

According to Professor Feder, the way to solve the political crowd-out dilemma is by changing the very nature of American culture. The focus on individualism must be replaced with a concern for the community and recognition that all Americans are part of a single community. "The challenge to improving or achieving universal coverage is to decide whether we are a society in which it is every man, woman or child for him/herself or one in which we are all in it together."[20(p464)] Clearly, the country remains divided about the extent to which "we are all in it together." Shortly before the ACA passed, over half of people surveyed (54%) said they would not be willing to pay more so others could have access to health insurance.[21] The continued debate over the future of the ACA has highlighted fundamental disagreements about how our health system should be structured and the proper role of individuals and governments in ensuring the country's good health.

▶ Unsuccessful Attempts to Pass National Health Insurance Reform

Since the early 1900s, when medical knowledge became advanced enough to make health care and health insurance desirable commodities, there have been periodic attempts to implement universal coverage through national health reform. The Socialist Party was the first U.S. political party to support health insurance in 1904, but the main engine behind early efforts for national reform was the American Association for Labor Legislation (AALL), a "social progressive" group that hoped to reform capitalism, not overthrow it.[22(p243)] In 1912, Progressive Party candidate Theodore Roosevelt supported a social insurance platform modeled on the European social insurance tradition that included health insurance, workers' compensation, old-age pensions, and unemployment insurance. After his loss to Woodrow Wilson, the national health insurance movement was without a strong national leader for three decades.

The AALL continued to support a form of health insurance after Roosevelt's defeat and drafted a model bill in 1915. This bill followed the European model, limiting participation to working class employees and their dependents. Benefits included medical aid, sick pay, maternity benefits, and a death benefit. These costs were to be financed by employers, employees, and the state. The AALL believed that health insurance for the working population would reduce poverty and increase society's productivity and well-being through healthier workers and citizens.

Opposition to AALL's bill came from several sources.[22(pp247–249)] Although some members of the American Medical Association (AMA) approved of the bill conceptually, physician support rapidly evaporated when details emerged about aspects of the plan that would negatively impact their income and autonomy. The American Federation of Labor (a labor union) opposed compulsory health insurance because it wanted workers to rely on their own economic strength, not the state, to obtain better wages and benefits. In addition, the federation was concerned that it would lose power if the government, not the union, secured benefits for workers. Employers were generally opposed to the bill, contending that supporting public health was a better way to ensure productivity. In addition, they feared that providing health insurance to employees might promote malingering instead of reducing lost workdays. After experiencing the high cost associated with workers' compensation, employers also were not eager to take on an additional expensive benefit. Of course, the part of the insurance industry that had already established a profitable niche in the death benefit business was strongly opposed to a bill that included a death benefit provision. Employers, healthcare providers, and insurers have, in general, remained staunch opponents of national health reform over the years, whereas unions have supported national reform efforts. However, this dynamic has changed recently with more provider groups, employers, and even some insurers calling for a national solution to the problems of rising healthcare costs and the uninsured.

The country's entry into World War I in 1917 also changed the health reform debate. Many physicians who supported the AALL bill entered the military, shifting their focus away from the domestic health policy debate. Anti-German sentiment was high, so opponents of the bill gained traction by denouncing compulsory health insurance as anti-American. One pamphlet read as follows: "What is Compulsory Social Health Insurance? It is a dangerous device, invented in Germany, announced by the German Emperor from the throne the same year he started plotting and preparing to conquer the world."[22(p253)]

The next time national health insurance might have taken hold was from the mid-1930s through the early 1940s as the country was coping with the difficulties of the Great Depression. During this time there was a significant increase in government programs, including the creation of Social Security in 1935, which provided old-age assistance, unemployment compensation, and public assistance. Yet the fourth prong of the social insurance package, health insurance, remained elusive. President Franklin Roosevelt heeded his staff's advice to leave health insurance out of Social Security because of the strong opposition it would create.[22(p267)] Opposition from the AMA was particularly strong—they believed that "socialized medicine" would increase bureaucracy, limit physician freedom, and interfere with the doctor–patient relationship.

Even so, members of Roosevelt's administration continued to push for national health insurance. The Interdepartmental Committee to Coordinate Health and Welfare Activities was created in 1935 and took on the task of studying the nation's healthcare needs. This job fell to its Technical Committee on Medical Care. Instead of supporting a federal program, the committee proposed subsidies to the states for operating health programs. Components of the proposal included expanding maternal and child health and public health programs under Social Security, expanding hospital construction, increasing aid for medical care for the indigent, studying a general medical care program, and creating a compensation program for those who lost wages due to disability.

Although President Roosevelt established a National Health Conference to discuss the recommendation, he never fully supported the medical care committee's proposal. With the success of conservatives in the 1938 election and the administration's concerns about fighting the powerful physician and state medical society lobbies, national health reform did not have a place on Roosevelt's priority list. Senator Robert Wagner (D-NY) introduced a bill that followed the committee's recommendations in 1939, and although it passed in the Senate, it did not garner support from the president or from the House.

World War II provided another opportunity for the opposition to label national health insurance as socialized medicine. But once the war neared an end, President Roosevelt finally called for an "economic bill of rights" that included medical care. President Truman picked up where Roosevelt left off, strongly advocating for national health insurance. President Truman's proposal included expanding hospitals, increasing public health and maternal and child health services, providing federal aid for medical research and education, and, for the first time, a single health insurance program for all.[22(p281)] Heeding lessons from earlier reform failures, Truman emphasized that his plan was not socialized medicine and that the delivery system for medical and hospital care would not change.

Again, there was strong opposition to the proposal. The AMA vehemently rejected the proposal, and most other healthcare groups opposed it as well. Although the public initially approved of it, there was no consensus about how national health insurance should be structured, and more people preferred modest voluntary plans over a national, compulsory, comprehensive health insurance program.[22(p282)] Additional opposition came from the American Bar Association, the Chamber of Commerce, and even some federal agencies concerned about losing control over their existing programs. In the end, only the hospital construction portion of the proposal was enacted.

When Truman won reelection on a national health insurance platform in 1948, it appeared the tide had turned. However, the AMA continued its strong opposition and its attempts to link national health insurance to socialism. Congress considered various compromises but never reached a consensus. The public remained uncertain about what kind of plan to favor. Employers maintained their opposition to compulsory insurance. In addition, one large group of potential supporters—veterans— was disinterested in the debate because they had already secured extensive medical coverage through the Veterans Administration. As the Korean War moved forward, Truman's focus shifted away from national health insurance and toward the war effort and other priorities.

National health insurance did not return to the national policy agenda until the 1970s. The landscape then was quite different from Truman's era. Medicaid and Medicare had been created, healthcare costs had begun to rise exponentially, and the economy was deteriorating. In 1969, President Nixon declared that a "massive crisis" existed in health care and that unless it was fixed immediately, the country's medical system would collapse.[22(p381)] The general public seemed to agree, with 75% of respondents in one survey concurring that the healthcare system was in crisis.[22(p381)] Democrats still controlled Congress by a significant margin, and Senator Edward Kennedy (D-MA) and Representative Martha Griffiths (D-MI), the first woman to serve on the powerful House Committee on Ways and Means, proposed a comprehensive, federally operated health insurance system.

At the same time, a movement supporting health care and patient rights was gaining momentum. These included rights to informed consent, to refuse treatment, to due process for involuntary commitment, and to equal access to health care.[22(p389)] The public was both anxious to obtain care and willing to challenge the authority of healthcare providers.

The Nixon administration's first attempt at health reform focused on changing the healthcare system's financing from one dominated by a fee-for-service system, which created incentives to provide more and more expensive services, to one that promoted restraint, efficiency, and the health of the patient. The result was a "health maintenance strategy" intended to stimulate the private industry to create health maintenance organizations (HMOs) through federal planning grants and loan guarantees, with the goal of enrolling 90% of the population in an HMO by the end of the 1970s.[22(pp395-396)] Ironically, group health plans, often labeled socialized medicine, had become the centerpiece of a Republican reform strategy.

Nixon's proposal included an employer mandate to provide a minimum package of benefits under a National Health Insurance Standards Act; a federally administered Family Health Insurance Program for low-income families that had a less generous benefit package than the one required by the National Health Insurance Standards Act; reductions in Medicare spending to help defray the costs; a call for an increase in the supply of physicians; and a change in how medical schools were subsidized. Opponents were plentiful, and this plan did not come to fruition. Some believed the plan was a gift to private insurance companies. Advocates for the poor were outraged at the second tier of benefits for low-income families. The AMA was concerned about HMOs interfering with physician practices and supported an alternative that provided tax credits for buying private insurance.

After the 1972 election, Nixon proposed a second plan that covered everyone and offered more comprehensive coverage. Private insurance companies would cover the employed and a government-run program would cover the rest of the population, with both groups receiving the same benefit package. Senator Kennedy and Representative Wilbur Mills (D-AR) supported a similar plan, and it appeared a compromise was close at hand. However, labor unions and liberal organizations preferred the original Kennedy plan and resisted compromising with the hope of gaining power in the 1974 post-Watergate elections. Fearing the same political shift, insurance companies actually supported a catastrophic insurance plan proposed by Senator Russell Long (D-LA), believing it was better than any plan that would come out of a more liberal Congress after the elections. Once again, there was no majority support for any of the bills, and a national health insurance plan was not enacted.

Although President Jimmy Carter gave lip service to national health reform, he never fully supported a proposal. It was not until the election of Bill Clinton in 1992 that the next real attempt at national health insurance was made. The Clinton administration plan, dubbed the Health Security Act, was designed to create national health insurance without spending new federal funds or shifting coverage from private to public insurance. It relied on the concept of "managed competition," which combined elements of managed care and market competition.

Under the Health Security Act, a National Health Board would have established national and regional spending limits and regulated premium increases. "Health alliances" would have included a variety of plans that were competing for the business of employees and unemployed citizens in each geographic area. All plans were to have a guaranteed scope of benefits and uniform cost-sharing. Employers would have been required to provide coverage for their workers at a defined high level of benefits, and those with 5,000 employees or fewer would have had to purchase plans through the health alliance. Subsidies were provided for low-income individuals and small businesses. Funding was to be provided from cost-containment measures that were reinvested. Forced by the Congressional Budget Office (CBO) to provide an alternative funding strategy should the cost containment not create enough funds, the plan also included the option of capping insurance premium growth and reducing provider payments.

Like the national health insurance plans before it, the Health Security Act had opponents from many directions. The health alliances were attacked as big government, employers resisted mandates and interference with their fringe benefits, some advocates feared that cost containment would lead to care rationing, the insured were concerned about losing some of their existing benefits or cost-sharing arrangements, the elderly feared losing Medicare, and academic health centers were concerned about losing funds based on new graduate medical education provisions.[22(p463)] In addition, the usually strong support from unions was missing because of an earlier disagreement with the president on trade matters. It is also generally accepted that the Clinton administration made several political mistakes that made a difficult political chore nearly impossible. The Health Security Act never made it to a vote.

▶ The Stars Align (Barely): How the Affordable Care Act Became Law

In many ways, 2010 was a very unlikely year to pass a national health reform plan. The country had been growing increasingly ideological, with the popular and electoral votes almost evenly split in both the 2000 and 2004 presidential elections. George W. Bush beat Al Gore despite losing the popular vote in 2000, and Bush beat John Kerry in 2004 with only 51% of the popular vote.[23] Even though Barack Obama won the electoral vote in a landslide over John McCain (365 to 173), only 53% of the population voted for Obama in 2008.[24]

In addition to the ideological divide, a financial crisis erupted toward the end of the 2008 presidential election. In October 2008, President Bush signed into law the Emergency Economic Stabilization Act, which included the $700 billion Troubled Asset Relief Program (TARP) that allowed the federal government to take over distressed assets, primarily bad mortgage loans, from private financial institutions.[25] It was argued that TARP was necessary to save the financial industry from collapsing, which could have led to another Great Depression. Even with TARP, the United States (and many other countries) entered into a recessionary period. Many individuals lived in homes they could no longer afford, banks limited lending opportunities, and employers laid off millions of workers due to the drop in consumer spending. In an effort to improve the economy, Obama signed into law the American Recovery and Reinvestment Act of 2009, also known as the stimulus bill.[26] This almost $800 billion effort was intended to save existing jobs, create new jobs, and spur long-term growth of the U.S. economy. Although TARP was not popular with politicians or the general public, it was seen as necessary by members of both political parties and signed into law by a Republican president. Unlike TARP, however, the stimulus bill was not a bipartisan effort. Republicans in the House unanimously opposed the stimulus bill and only three Republicans voted for the bill in the Senate.

Not surprisingly, health care was not the only issue on voters' minds during the election campaign. Shortly before the election, 43% of registered voters ranked the economy as their number one priority. Economic concerns trumped health care, which ranked second, by an almost two-to-one margin.[27] Although voters from both political parties ranked the economy as their top priority, differences emerged along party lines regarding the next most important issue. Democratic voters ranked health care second, whereas both Republican and Independent voters were more concerned about the size and power of the federal government. These results were not surprising; Democrats have ranked health care as a higher priority than Republican and Independent voters in every presidential election from 1988 to 2012.[28(p2053)]

It was against this backdrop of a faltering economy, partisan differences, and the recent passage of two massive government spending bills that President Obama pursued a national health reform plan. Given the history of failed reform efforts, it would have been an accomplishment to pass health reform in the best of times, and clearly this was not the best of times. How did Obama and the 111th Congress succeed? It was a combination of having commitment, exhibiting leadership, applying lessons from past failures, and being pragmatic that lead to the passage of health reform.

Commitment and Leadership

It is highly unlikely that the 2010 health reform effort would have succeeded without a passionate and committed president willing to make health reform a priority. Health care has long been a priority for Democrats, and President Obama was no exception. Perhaps Obama's dedication to passing health reform stemmed in part from his personal experience: Obama's mother died of ovarian cancer, and he had seen her worry about paying her medical bills as much as beating the disease.[29] Thus, for Obama, signing comprehensive health reform legislation into law would represent the opportunity to make sure that others would not endure the same experience.

Some of Obama's political advisors suggested waiting to tackle health reform until after taking action to address the poor economy and rising unemployment. Even voters who supported Obama were split over what his priorities should be during his first days in office.[30] Just days before the election, Obama suggested that the economy and energy independence were higher priorities than health reform. To Obama, that meant he should tackle several majors issues at once, not put health reform on the back burner.

Health reform efforts did not begin smoothly. President Obama initially wanted former U.S. senator Tom Daschle to run both the Department of Health and Human Services (HHS) and the White House Office on Health Reform. It was thought that his experience in the Senate and relationships with legislators were the right combination to take the lead on health reform. When his nomination was derailed due to personal tax problems, it was not a good omen. As deliberations in Congress lagged, Democrats were not able to present a bill to President Obama before recessing for the summer. During the summer of 2009, members of Congress went home to their constituents and held town hall meetings to discuss health reform. Some of the meetings erupted in vocal opposition to health reform, and the media focused on these town hall meetings throughout the summer. Obama and the Democrats were criticized for losing the momentum for reform by letting the debate linger.

At the same time, there were several instances when the health reform effort appeared politically doomed, and President Obama's leadership made a clear difference. Obama attempted to reclaim the upper hand on health reform with a speech to a joint session of Congress in September 2009. He memorably proclaimed, "I am not the first president to take up health reform, but I intend to be the last."[31] Although public support for health reform had been on the decline for several months, September 2009 polls showed that 62% still thought it was important to address health reform at that time, and 53% thought the country as a whole would be better off if health reform passed.[32] Less support existed for the Democrats' specific reform proposal, however, with 46% in support of the proposed change and 48% opposed to it.[33]

In January 2010, an event occurred that some assumed was the death knell of health reform. In the 2008 elections, Democrats had made significant gains in Congress, earning a 59–41 majority in the Senate and a 257–178 majority in the House. Furthermore, Senator Arlen Specter of Pennsylvania switched parties, giving Democrats the crucial 60th vote needed for a filibuster-proof majority. Although the numbers were now in their favor, President Obama, Senate Majority Leader Harry Reid (D-NV), and House Speaker Nancy Pelosi (D-CA) would have to balance the competing interests of conservative Democrats who were concerned with having too much government intervention, progressive Democrats who sought a public insurance option to compete with private companies, Blue Dog Democrats who were most concerned with fiscal discipline, and pro-life and pro-choice factions who would battle over whether and how abortion services would be included in any health reform bill.

Then, in August 2009, Senator Ted Kennedy (D-MA) died. In office for 47 years, Kennedy was not only a lifelong supporter of health reform but also an expert negotiator who could work with Republicans and possibly achieve a bipartisan consensus. The January 2010 special election to fill his seat was won by Republican Scott Brown, who campaigned against the Democrats' health reform plan. In a post-election poll, 42% of voters said they voted for Brown to stop health reform from moving ahead.[34]

Despite this setback and concerns by some that health reform efforts should be abandoned, Obama, along with Reid and Pelosi, remained strong in his conviction to pursue reform. President Obama's senior advisors said it would be a "terrible mistake" to walk away from the process based on Brown's victory, and Pelosi reminded her caucus how detrimental it was when Democrats abandoned the health reform effort during the Clinton administration.[35] In his State of the Union address just a week after Senator Brown claimed the special election, President Obama tied his health reform efforts to fixing the economy and reiterated his commitment to the issue:

> And it is precisely to relieve the burden on middle class families that we still need health reform. Now let's be clear, I did not choose to tackle this issue to get some legislative victory under my belt. And by now it should be fairly obvious that I didn't take on health reform because it was good

politics.... Here is what I ask of Congress though: Do not walk away from reform. Not now. Not when we are so close. Let us find a way to come together and finish the job for the American people.[36]

Obama was not alone in providing leadership on health reform. Reid's and Pelosi's determination to see health reform succeed, and their skill in mobilizing and controlling their caucuses, were essential to the passage of the ACA. It is likely that health reform would not have passed without the skillful efforts of all three leaders working together. Even so, it is clear that the health reform effort would not even have begun without a president who put health reform at the top of the agenda and stuck with it despite the pitfalls and political opposition.

Lessons from Failed Health Reform Efforts

The Obama administration tried to avoid events that doomed earlier health reform efforts. Although the failed effort by the Clinton administration probably provided the most relevant lessons, Obama confronted some of the same obstacles that reformers had faced decades earlier. At times, President Obama was accused of learning some of the lessons too well, swinging the pendulum too far to the other side. Although that debate may continue, clearly the way in which the Obama administration applied those lessons brought him success where others had failed before him.

President Clinton was criticized for not moving quickly enough to try to enact health reform after he was elected in 1992. He did not present a plan to Congress until a year into his presidency, having been sidetracked by other issues such as the economy, including a budget showdown with Republicans, and whether gays should be allowed to serve in the military. Even after he finally sent his healthcare proposal to Congress, Clinton was preoccupied with other issues that sapped his political capital, such as passing the North American Free Trade Agreement and the fallout from the deaths of 18 American soldiers in Somalia.

President Obama, over the objection of some aides, chose to address health reform as quickly as possible, despite also having to tackle the poor economy and possible collapse of the financial sector. Obama was elected into office with a 70% approval rating, and he moved to capitalize on his popularity.[37] It was almost inevitable that his approval rating would decline as he tried to turn the promise of a campaign into the reality of running the country. As Lyndon Johnson said after winning the 1964 election in a landslide, "Every day while I'm in office, I'm gonna lose votes."[38(p172)] In addition, it is almost universally expected that the president's party will lose seats in the midterm elections. From 2000 to 2010, the incumbent party lost an average of 18.5 seats in the House and 2.5 seats in the Senate.[39(p1097)] Obama was correct to assume his Democratic majorities in Congress would not last long. After the 2010 midterm elections the Democrats lost control of the House and several seats in the Senate.

President Obama also dealt with interest groups in a different way from his predecessors. Previous failed efforts at health reform have shown that those vested interests can be important players in the debate. In general, though not in all instances, provider groups, insurers, and employers have opposed health reform, whereas unions have supported health reform efforts. All of these stakeholders have been known to devote significant resources and apply pressure on their representatives to support their point of view. During its reform effort, the Clinton administration warred with many stakeholder groups, with insurance companies and small businesses taking a leading role.[18]

Obama took a different approach than Clinton by making deals with various stakeholders at the outset of the health reform debate. The lure of millions of newly insured customers helped convince the Pharmaceutical Research and Manufacturers of America and the American Hospital Association to contribute to health reform financing through reduced Medicare and Medicaid payments. In addition, the health insurance industry supported universal insurance coverage under health reform. After being credited with helping derail the Clinton health plan, the Health Insurance Association of America favored the general idea of health reform, though it differed with Obama and the Democrats on some of the specifics. To be fair, Clinton may not have been able to broker deals with these stakeholders in the 1990s no matter how hard he tried. A combination of a changing healthcare environment, the likelihood that some type of health reform was likely to pass, and the uncertain future of employer-sponsored insurance made it more palatable for interest groups to try to influence instead of oppose the 2010 legislation.[40]

Clinton was also criticized for failing to master the legislative process. The Clinton administration chose to design the health reform plan itself and developed a complicated and secretive process, headlined by the Health Care Task Force run by Hillary Clinton, to do so. Although naming Hillary Clinton as the leader of the task force signaled the administration's commitment to the issue, she became a lightning rod for criticism, and questions about the appropriateness of the First Lady taking on such a significant policy role detracted from the substance of the health reform debate. Instead of negotiating with Congress, the administration debated the specifics of health reform among its own advisors and then asked Congress to pass the bill they had developed. Shutting out members of Congress instead of negotiating with them and taking over Congress's role in developing legislation was not, it turned out, a formula for success.

President Obama learned from Clinton's mistakes as well as from other presidents' legislative achievements. Instead of presenting a detailed plan or written legislation to Congress, success has often been found in outlining ideas and principles and letting Congress work through the details. When President Johnson was trying to get a Medicare bill passed, he told key members of Congress that he would not delve into the details of the bill but generally pushed for a larger package. When President George W. Bush was pursuing a new Medicare prescription drug benefit, he outlined his desire for an approach that worked with the private sector and encouraged competition, but let Congress find the exact formula that would pass.[39(p1097)]

Similarly, Obama set out his principles but left the work of drafting a bill and fleshing out the details to Congress. On June 2, 2009, President Obama sent a letter to Senators Kennedy and Baucus, two leaders in the health reform effort, outlining his "core belief" that Americans deserved better and more affordable health insurance choices and that a health reform bill must not add to the federal deficit.[41] Although he let the negotiators know what his priorities were, Obama stayed above the fray during the legislative process. Whereas he preferred a public option to compete with private insurers, he did not insist on it. Although Obama campaigned against an individual mandate as a presidential candidate, he was open to including it in the bill. The president refused to be drawn into the debate over taxing generous health plans or creating a Medicare cost-containment commission. Instead, he focused his efforts on persuading Congress not to give up on the effort, bringing together various factions of the Democratic caucus, and reaching out to the public to garner support for health reform.

The legislative process for completing the bill was long, rocky, and ultimately partisan. The House of Representatives moved more quickly and with less fractious debate than the Senate. Instead of having multiple House committees work on competing bills, as occurred during the Clinton administration, House Democratic leaders created a "Tri-Committee" bill jointly sponsored by Charles Rangel (D-NY), Henry Waxman (D-CA), and George Miller (D-CA), the chairmen of the House Ways and Means, Energy and Commerce, and Education and Labor (later renamed the Education and Workforce committee) committees, respectively. On November 7, 2009, the House passed its health reform bill with only two votes to spare, 220–215.[42] Only one Republican voted for it, and 39 conservative Democrats voted against it. The bill from the then-more-liberal House contained several provisions that were likely to be rejected by the Senate: a public health insurance option to compete with private plans, a national health insurance exchange instead of state-based exchanges, more generous subsidies for low-income individuals, a broader expansion of Medicaid, and higher taxes on wealthier Americans.

Finance Committee Chairman Max Baucus (D-MT) led the effort in the Senate. The legislative process he established was lengthy, and some observers believed he compromised on too many issues in an attempt to forge a bipartisan bill. For a time Senator Charles Grassley (R-IA) actively participated in the health reform deliberations, and a few other Republican senators appeared willing to consider a bipartisan measure. Ultimately, however, a bipartisan agreement could not be reached. In a 2009 Christmas Eve vote, the Baucus bill passed 60–39, with all Democrats and two Independents voting for the measure and all Republicans voting against it.[43]

Shortly after the New Year, members of the House and Senate began meeting to resolve differences between the bills passed in the House and the Senate. Before those differences were resolved, however, Scott Brown was elected to fill Kennedy's seat in the Senate and the Democrats no longer had a filibuster-proof majority. Before the special election that led to Brown's victory, it was assumed that after the Senate passed a health reform measure, House and Senate negotiators would work out their differences in a conference committee, with each chamber then voting to pass the compromise bill. With Brown's election and his opposition to health reform, however, this plan became unworkable. Democratic congressional leaders were left with few options, all of them unpalatable: the House could pass the Senate version of the bill; Democrats could try to use the reconciliation process—which does not allow for the use of filibusters and only requires a simple majority vote—to pass a new comprehensive bill; the House and Senate could compromise on a much smaller, more incremental health reform bill that focused on areas where a bipartisan agreement could be reached; or Democrats could abandon their efforts to pass a health reform bill. The day after Brown's election, House Speaker Pelosi appeared to eliminate the easiest (legislatively speaking) of these paths by declaring that the House would not pass the Senate version of the bill: "I don't think it's possible to pass the Senate bill in the House. I don't see the votes for it at this time."[44]

In the end, a compromise was reached. House and Senate leaders agreed to use the budget reconciliation process to amend the Senate bill. The House then passed the Senate version of the bill along with a companion reconciliation bill that amended certain aspects of the Senate bill. The reconciliation bill included more generous subsidies for individuals to purchase insurance than existed in the stand-alone Senate bill, the closure of the Medicare Part D doughnut hole, a tax on more generous insurance plans, changes to the penalties on individuals who would not buy insurance and for employers that would not offer insurance, and an increase in Medicare and investment taxes for higher earners. The Senate then passed the reconciliation bill. Once again, the final vote to approve the bills was along party lines. The House approved the Senate bill by a vote of 219–212, with all Republicans and 34 Democrats voting against it.[45] President Obama signed the bill into law on March 23, 2010.[1]

Some observers argue that Obama may have overlearned the lesson about working with Congress and that in doing so he did not provide enough guidance to legislators and allowed the debate over health reform to linger for too long.[39(p1097)] On the one hand, it is difficult to criticize Obama's approach because he was ultimately successful. On the other hand, could the problems stemming from the 2009 town halls and Scott Brown's election have been avoided, and would public opinion of the health reform effort be higher, if the process had been better managed? Only time will tell whether Obama was successful over the long term (e.g., Is the law effective? Will the public support it over time? Will it be repealed?) and whether the political cost of the lengthy battle hurt the Democrats more than passing the bill helped them.

Political Pragmatism

President Obama is both credited and criticized for being as pragmatic as necessary to help ensure that a health reform law came to fruition. He was comfortable making deals with industry stakeholders even though those agreements limited the savings and other changes that could have been achieved in the health reform bill. Obama ultimately signed a bill that did not include a public option, even though he preferred that one be included, and his liberal base thought health reform without such an option was not true reform. An argument over abortion nearly derailed the bill in its final days, and Obama supported a compromise on abortion language to keep enough Democrats in the fold. Even his goal of creating universal insurance coverage was not recognized. Yet Obama's willingness to be pragmatic instead of staunchly principled, taking some victories instead of an all-or-nothing approach, allowed him to succeed in passing a health reform bill where others had failed.[40(p1116)] Some people argued it was worse to pass a flawed bill than not pass a bill at all, but Obama believed the promise of reducing the uninsured rate and gaining numerous health insurance market reforms were worth the compromises he made.

▶ Overview of the Patient Protection and Affordable Care Act

As noted earlier, while President Obama left the details of health reform legislation to Congress, he did lay out what he believed to be the most important principles that should guide the legislation's development. Soon after becoming president in 2009,

Obama delineated those principles, saying that any health reform measure should do the following:

1. Protect families' financial health (slowing the growth of out-of-pocket expenses and protecting people from bankruptcy due to catastrophic illness)
2. Make health insurance coverage more affordable (reducing administrative costs, wiping out unnecessary tests and services, limiting insurers' ability to charge higher premiums for certain populations)
3. Aim for insurance coverage universality
4. Provide portability of insurance coverage
5. Guarantee choice of health plans and providers (including keeping current ones)
6. Invest in disease prevention and wellness initiatives
7. Improve patient safety and healthcare quality
8. Maintain long-term fiscal sustainability (reducing cost growth, improving productivity, adding new revenue sources)

The extent to which these principles were brought to life in what eventually became the Affordable Care Act lives along a spectrum: for example, health insurance was absolutely made more affordable for millions of people; disease prevention and wellness initiatives seem to be gaining momentum, though slowly; and universal insurance coverage was absolutely not achieved. Whatever the case with any particular principle, it is instructive to look to four key reforms that became law under the ACA as having paved the way for President Obama's overall vision to come to fruition. These four reforms essentially reordered long-standing relationships among health system stakeholders (individuals, providers, insurers, employers, governments, etc.). As a result of this reordering, all of these stakeholders were legally obligated to alter normative behaviors.

The first major change, known as the individual mandate, is a requirement that individuals maintain "minimum essential health coverage" (i.e., health insurance) or face financial penalties that are spelled out in the ACA. This requirement was a critically important beam in the ACA architecture: because it creates a new, large pool of individuals who will be paying premiums to insurance companies, it created leverage for policymakers who were eager for the private insurers to accept many of the ACA's other insurance reforms that may otherwise have been unpalatable. For certain individuals whose socioeconomic status makes it impossible for them to purchase (or gain through an employer) the type of minimum coverage mandated by the ACA, and who do not qualify for Medicaid (even under the ACA expansion), federal subsidies are made available under the law.

The second fundamental change results from reforms that prohibit or curtail existing health insurer and health plan practices (these are the types of reforms, noted in the preceding paragraph, that all insurers—not just those who sell products through the new exchanges, described in the following paragraph—were forced to accept to reciprocate for the new group of premium payers they would insure as a result of the individual mandate). For example, the ACA prohibits insurers from considering an applicant's preexisting conditions when determining whether to insure the applicant, guarantees the renewability of an individual's existing insurance plan, requires insurers to cover certain preventive and immunization services, and guarantees coverage for dependent children who are 26 years old or younger.

The third key change is the creation of health insurance "exchanges" or "marketplaces" in each state. These are essentially online shopping sites, the purpose of which is to make it easier for individuals and small employers to compare and purchase health insurance. Because the ACA requires everyone to carry health insurance, and because the insurance marketplace has not historically been easy to navigate, policymakers forced the creation of regulated state-based exchanges to help with the purchase of individual and small-group insurance plans.

The final major reform is an expansion of the existing Medicaid program. This reform has the potential to dramatically increase the number of individuals who can gain access to insurance coverage—and thus access to better and more appropriate health care. Because states cannot be forced to implement this expansion (more on this to follow in the discussion of the U.S. Supreme Court's decision around the constitutionality of the ACA), and many states have thus far declined to implement the expansion, this potential has yet to become a reality. Although the ACA does not completely alter the way health insurance is provided by, say, establishing a single-payer system or even a large government-run insurance plan to compete with private insurers, the law does make significant philosophical and practical changes in how health insurance is regulated, structured, and administered. Indeed, as a result of the reforms and reordering just described, recent estimates indicate that the ACA has resulted in 20 million people gaining insurance, dropping the uninsured rate from 16% in 2010 to a historically low 9.1% in early 2016.[46] In addition, as a result of the essential health benefits requirement, there is a large segment of the population that is no longer underinsured because of insurance plans that do not offer comprehensive benefits.

Even so, many people contend that the ACA falls short in its reform of the healthcare delivery system. And in many cases they are correct. The ACA is most notable for the transformations it makes to health insurance—both access to it and its content—rather than for structural reforms made to the delivery system. Many provisions that focus on improving the healthcare delivery system, increasing the quality of care received by patients, reducing healthcare costs, and incentivizing providers to reconsider traditional methods of delivering care, often exist in the form of temporary pilot programs that may never be enacted permanently even if they prove to be valuable. Other analysts contend that these provisions were written as strongly as they could be at the time given the political environment and data available to policymakers. According to this view, the ACA provides the secretary of the U.S. Department of Health and Human Services with unprecedented authority to make the pilot programs permanent, and it would have been irresponsible to implement more permanent, wholesale changes without more evidence. In any case, as sweeping as the ACA is, it is far from being the last step that needs to be taken to improve how health care is provided in the United States. We turn now to a more detailed discussion of the ACA's key components.

Individual Mandate

An individual mandate is a requirement that individuals purchase health insurance. This is not a new idea. President Clinton proposed an individual mandate in 1993 as part of his Health Security Act, and other competing proposals at the time, including those supported by Republicans, also included an individual mandate. Massachusetts, the only state in the country to require that everyone over age 18 have health insurance, included an individual mandate as one way to achieve that goal. Switzerland and the Netherlands also included an individual mandate in their health reform plans.[47] During the 2008 election, Obama originally supported a mandate for children to be covered but suggested waiting to see if a mandate was necessary for adults after implementing other major health reform changes.

While the individual mandate is not a new idea and has been championed by both Republicans and Democrats at different times in history, it has proven to be a politically perilous route to reducing the number of uninsured. Opposition to the individual mandate has softened over time, but public opinion remains split and partisan. A 2017 poll taken during the debate about the Republican ACA repeal and replacement efforts found that 50% of respondents supported retaining the individual mandate, while 48% preferred to eliminate this provision.[48] This represents a shift in favor of the mandate over a 2013 poll that found 58% of respondents opposed.[49] Over half of Republicans (55%) opposed the individual mandate in 2017 as compared to 84% in 2013. Democrats remained supportive of the individual mandated with 60% preferring to keep the mandate in place in 2017, similar to the 57% who felt that way in 2013.[48]

It appears that some individuals do not prefer to be told they have to purchase health insurance by the government, even if it is a choice they made on their own prior to the passage of the ACA. But issues such as affordability or difficulty using the federal exchange website were more likely to be cited as reasons for not having health insurance than political opposition to the mandate. A poll conducted shortly after the first enrollment period closed found that most people who remained uninsured cited affordability (39%) or job-related reasons (22%), while only 9% felt they did not want or need health insurance.[50] Understandably, affordability remains a top issue for the public. In a recent poll, all respondents (regardless of political leanings) ranked limiting the amount individuals pay for health care as their top priority.[51] Almost half (49%) were very worried or somewhat worried about not being able to afford health care services in the future.[51]

Individual mandates can be set up in a variety of ways, but usually individuals who do not comply will be required to pay some sort of penalty. The penalty is intended to provide both an incentive to comply with the law and to raise funds to cover the cost of health care for those individuals who choose not to carry health insurance. Individual mandates are considered to be a cornerstone of health reform efforts because they ensure that everyone covered by the mandate will be in an insurance pool to help cover costs and share risk.

The mandate is considered essential because without it people who are in poor health or otherwise expect to use more healthcare services will be more likely to purchase health insurance, whereas healthier people will be more likely to opt out of insurance coverage. This would lead to an insurance pool that is relatively sick and thus more expensive, a problem referred to as *adverse selection*. For example, the Congressional Budget Office (CBO) estimated that the House Republican ACA replacement bill would result in 16 million fewer insured people by 2019, mostly due to the elimination of the individual mandate.[52] Removing the penalties for being uninsured and the resulting higher premiums would lead many individuals to drop their insurance coverage.

Due to fears of adverse selection, analysts have been closely watching how many young people (ages 18–34), who are more likely to be healthy, have signed up for health insurance. While ideally 40% of enrollees would be in this age range in order to prevent adverse selection, only about 28% of the 8 million enrollees signed up at the end of the first enrollment period in April 2014 were young adults.[53] About 45% of taxpayers who either paid a penalty for not having insurance or claimed an exemption from the mandate that year were under 35.[54] While still well below the target level, the number of enrollees under age 35 doubled from 2014 to 2015 and the Obama administration prioritized young adult enrollment in subsequent years.[55]

The individual mandate is also an essential feature of health reform because healthy individuals who choose not to purchase health insurance but then later need health care will likely receive some care even though they are uninsured. This is especially true if the individuals have the resources to pay for healthcare services. These individuals are referred to as *free riders* because they avoid paying premiums for health insurance during their healthy years but then enjoy the benefits of healthcare services when they become sick. In 2015 over 7 million people who earned more than $75,000 were uninsured.[56] Because it is likely that many of these individuals could have afforded to purchase health insurance, some analysts consider this evidence of the free-rider problem.[47]

Beyond the issues of adverse selection and free riders, the individual mandate is considered essential to the architecture of the ACA because it was the carrot (in the form of new premium dollars) that enticed health insurers to support health reform. Starting in 2014 the ACA's individual mandate required that almost everyone purchase health insurance or pay a penalty. This penalty is phased in over time, beginning at the greater of $95 or 1% of taxable income per person in 2014 and growing to the greater of $695 or 2.5% of taxable income per person in 2016 and 2017. In subsequent years, the penalty amount increases through cost of living adjustments. The maximum penalty is the cost of the national average bronze plan sold through the marketplace. Some supporters of the mandate are concerned that the penalty is not large enough to incentivize individuals to purchase insurance because it would be much cheaper to pay the penalty.

There are a number of exceptions to the individual mandate requirement. Individuals are exempt from purchasing insurance if their income is below the tax-filing threshold (in 2016 this was $10,350 for single people under age 65 and $20,700 for couples under age 65), the lowest-cost plan option exceeds 8% of their income, they qualify for a religious exemption, they are incarcerated, they are undocumented immigrants, they were without coverage for less than 3 months, they are Native Americans, or they qualify as having a hardship. Based on a June 2013 HHS rule, hardship exemptions must be granted for individuals who experience an event that resulted in an unexpected increase in expenses such that purchasing health insurance would make it impossible to pay for necessities, such as food and shelter. The rule cites circumstances that would be considered under this exemption: homelessness, eviction, domestic violence, death of a close family member, bankruptcy, substantial recent medical debt, and disasters that substantially changed the individual's property.[57] Hardship exemptions are also allowed for individuals who would have qualified for Medicaid had their state chosen to expand the program under the ACA. There are additional hardship exemptions based on projected low income.[58] Some have criticized the exemptions for being so broad as to swallow the individual mandate.

To some, the individual mandate remains controversial. In addition to believing that it represents unwarranted government intrusion into private decision making, opponents of the individual mandate argued after the ACA was passed that Congress did not have the legal authority to impose such a requirement. This argument is grounded in jurisprudence relating to the federal Constitution's Commerce Clause, which gives Congress the power to "regulate commerce with foreign nations, and among the several states, and with the Indian tribes."[59] Since the 1940s the Supreme Court has interpreted the Commerce Clause to permit Congress to regulate economic activity that carries across state lines or that are local concerns that substantially affect interstate commerce, and several Commerce Clause cases have allowed the regulation of individual conduct (for example, the Supreme Court has upheld laws that prohibit an individual from refusing to interact with a minority and those that regulate an individual's ability to grow wheat or marijuana for home consumption[60]), and the regulation of health insurance has also been deemed within the scope of the Commerce Clause.[61]

Notwithstanding these cases, those who argued against the individual mandate contended that the Commerce Clause does not permit Congress to require an individual to purchase a service or good such as health insurance. In other words, the argument goes, an individual's decision not to purchase health insurance cannot be considered "economic activity" that Congress may regulate. Instead, it is argued, Congress is trying to regulate economic *in*activity—the decision not to purchase health insurance—and that this is not permitted under the Commerce Clause.[62]

On the other hand, those who contend the Commerce Clause permits Congress to establish an individual mandate to purchase health insurance argue that everyone uses healthcare services at some point in their lives. Decisions regarding health insurance are an economic activity because no one can opt out of the healthcare market—the decision individuals make is not whether to participate but how to participate in it. People will participate by purchasing health insurance now to cover the cost of future services or by paying out of pocket later at the time services are needed.

In the end, the Supreme Court upheld the individual mandate as a valid exercise of congressional *taxing* power; the court did, however, agree with those who maintained that the mandate was not permitted under the Commerce Clause. This outcome is described more fully later, when we provide an overview of the Supreme Court's June 2012 ruling on the constitutionality of the ACA.

BOX 1 Discussion Questions

Are there alternatives to the individual mandate that accomplish the same goals without engendering so much political turmoil? Could policymakers have designed an incentive system that would be as effective as a mandate? What are the pros and cons of using a mandate versus an incentive? Can you think of incentives to encourage enrollment that have occurred in other parts of the healthcare system?

State Health Insurance Exchanges/Marketplaces

The ACA established a new series of entities called health insurance exchanges (also referred to as marketplaces in federal documents) that are intended to create a more organized and competitive market for purchasing health insurance.[63] These exchanges are state-based and geared toward those who purchase health insurance as individuals (through American Health Benefit Exchanges) or through small businesses (through the Small Business Health Options Program, or SHOP).

The SHOP exchange struggled from the start with implementation delays and much lower than anticipated enrollment.[64] The Trump administration recently announced a rule that will effectively end the federally-facilitated SHOP exchange as of January 2018.[65] The small employer tax credit will remain in place, but businesses will purchase SHOP-qualified plans directly from insurers instead of on the exchange. According to the new rule, Centers for Medicare and Medicaid Services (CMS) will be working to find more efficient and effective ways to increase insurance coverage for small business employees.

Starting in 2014, the exchanges for individuals began offering a variety of health insurance plans that meet ACA criteria regarding plan benefits, payments, and consumer information. The Congressional Budget Office (CBO) projects that by 2027, 13 million individuals will purchase their own health insurance through an exchange.[66] This is significantly lower than earlier CBO estimates. Much of the difference is because fewer individuals are now projected to purchase unsubsidized plans on the exchange instead of directly from insurers in the nongroup market.[67] In addition, because fewer employers than anticipated dropped their employee coverage, CBO overestimated the number of individuals who would shift from employer coverage to marketplace plans.[68, 69]

The exchanges are a critical component of health reform because it would be untenable to require individuals to purchase health insurance without also making comprehensive and affordable health insurance options available. Individuals often face expensive and less comprehensive health insurance choices because their insurance pools are not extensive enough that the premiums paid by healthy individuals offset the costs associated with sicker ones. The exchanges are intended to create a new market by bringing together large numbers of individuals to create wider insurance pools. Individuals are eligible to purchase health insurance through an exchange if they live in the state where the exchange operates, are U.S. citizens or legal immigrants, and are not incarcerated. Additional requirements must be met, however, to obtain subsidies that reduce the cost of health insurance. Subsidies are available to individuals who meet the previously mentioned requirements and who also do not have access to affordable (as defined by the ACA) employer-sponsored insurance, meet specified income requirements, file taxes jointly (if married), and are not eligible for Medicaid, Medicare, or CHIP.[70]

Under the ACA, states have three main options when it came to exchanges: they can build their own, enter into a partnership with the federal government, or ignore the process altogether and thus default into what is referred to as a federally facilitated marketplace (FFM; this federally facilitated exchange was mandated by the ACA for states that were not willing or able to establish a state exchange or a partnership exchange). In a state-run exchange, the state either handles all functions or may use the federal IT platform; in a partnership exchange, states may administer plan management functions, in-person consumer assistance functions, or both, with HHS performing remaining responsibilities; and in the FFM, HHS performs all functions. Whatever the structure, the exchanges for individuals were required to be up and running by January 1, 2014. At the time of this writing, the breakdown is as follows: 16 states and the District of Colombia built their own exchange (with 5 of the states using the federal IT platform); 6 set up partnership exchanges; and 28 states defaulted to the FFM.[71] States also may form a regional exchange with other states or allow multiple exchanges within one state as long as each exchange covers a distinct geographical area. In addition, the federal Office of Personnel Management is required to offer at least two multistate plans within each exchange to provide individuals and businesses with additional choices.

The ACA requires the exchanges to ensure that plans meet other requirements of participating in the exchange. These requirements relate to marketing practices, provider networks, outreach and enrollment, following insurance market regulations, and providing information in plain language. In addition, the entity running the exchange must provide a call center for customers, maintain a website, develop uniform applications, provide information regarding eligibility for public programs, assist individuals in calculating their tax credits, and certify individuals who are exempt from the individual mandate requirement.

BOX 2 Provider Networks

An emerging policy and care delivery issue has been the question of whether provider networks available in plans offered in the exchanges are adequate. Prior to the ACA, insurers could control costs through a variety of mechanisms, including limiting benefits, excluding consumers with preexisting conditions, and using medical underwriting to charge higher premiums to higher risk individuals and groups. Plans would compete with each other based on price, benefits, cost-sharing, and other features. The ACA includes a variety of rules that eliminate these options, such as prohibition of exclusions based on preexisting conditions, guaranteed issue requirements, community rating requirements, essential health benefit requirements, and actuarial tiering of plans. As a result of ACA restrictions, many plans are trying to control costs by limiting provider networks and/or provider reimbursement. Of course, some providers may choose not to participate in exchange plans if the reimbursement is not sufficient.

Many consumers who purchase plans in an exchange choose plans based on the premium price and indicate they would prefer cheaper plans with narrow networks as opposed to expensive plans with broader networks. On the other hand, consumers who purchase plans through employer-sponsored insurance often prefer broader networks, even if the coverage is more expensive. Complaints about narrow networks range from consumers being disappointed that their usual doctor or local hospital is not in network, to questions about access to care, network transparency, and quality of care. Several lawsuits have been filed against plans regarding network transparency and provider terminations. In 2014 the Office of the Insurance Commissioner issued federal rules regarding network adequacy in individual and small-group plans, and CMS continues to issue guidance regarding network adequacy for Qualified Health Plans. State responses to network adequacy concerns have spanned the gamut, from Massachusetts requiring plans to develop tiered and narrow networks to promote cost savings, to several failed attempts by state legislatures to pass "any willing provider" laws that require insurers to include any provider willing to accept the insurers terms.

Essential Health Benefit Requirement

All Qualified Health Plans (QHP) that participate in an exchange (as well as individual and small-group plans outside of the exchanges) must offer a standard benefit package called essential health benefits (EHB) (**TABLE 1**).[72]

This represents the first time private health insurance plans are subject to a federal standard regarding what benefits must be offered. The ACA requires the secretary of HHS to ensure the scope of benefits is equal to the benefit level found in a "typical employer plan." Plans may not design their benefit or reimbursement packages in ways that discriminate based on age, disability, or expected length of life.[73]

While the ACA outlines 10 categories of services that must be provided in the essential health benefits package, the federal regulatory process left states with significant discretion about how they implemented this requirement. States had a choice of 10 federally approved health plans to serve as a benchmark to determine the breadth of the services covered under the EHB categories. These approved benchmark plans include the largest three small-group plans available in the state, the largest three state-employee health plans in the state, the largest three Federal Employee Health Benefit Program plan options for federal employees, or the state's

---

TABLE 1 Essential Health Benefits

All plans in the state exchanges must offer the following benefits:

- Ambulatory patient services

- Emergency services

- Hospitalization

- Maternity and newborn care

- Mental health services and substance use disorder services, including behavioral health treatment

- Prescription drugs

- Rehabilitative and habilitative services and devices (rehabilitative therapies improve, maintain, or prevent deterioration of functions that have been acquired [e.g., after an adult has surgery], whereas habilitative therapies are provided to achieve functions and skills never acquired [e.g., as with a developmentally disabled child])

- Laboratory services

- Prevention and wellness services and chronic disease management services

- Pediatric services, including vision and dental services

largest commercial HMO.[72] States that did not choose a benchmark plan were defaulted to the largest small-group plan offered in that state. Whether by choice or default, most states are using small-group plans, which are often less generous than large-group plans, as their benefit benchmark.[74]

In addition to using different benchmark plans across the country, in most states health insurers are allowed to substitute benefits *within* an EHB category, as long as the substitution is actuarially equivalent to the benefit it is replacing. For example, the benchmark plan might cover a blood screen for ovarian cancer, but the insurer could replace that laboratory test with coverage of a different, but actuarially equivalent, laboratory test.[72] Substitutes cannot occur across EHB categories (e.g., a lab test may not be substituted for a pediatric vision service), and substitution is not permitted for prescription drugs. Nine states and the District of Columbia prohibited this type of substitution in 2014.[72]

Further variation across the states may occur with habilitative service coverage and state benefit mandates. Habilitative services assist individuals with gaining or maintaining functional skills (e.g., speaking, walking). Prior to ACA passage, coverage for and the definition of habilitative services varied significantly. As part of ACA implementation, federal regulators permitted states to use the habilitative services definition in their benchmark plan (if there was such coverage), create their own coverage definition, or let the insurers define the coverage benefit.[72] As a result, the definition of habilitative services may differ across states and within states. Finally, some states passed laws that required insurers in their states to cover a particular benefit, such as obesity management services. Any benefit mandates that were in place before 2012 were incorporated into that state's EHB package, meaning the variation that was in place prior to health reform is likely to continue. It is less likely that states will add new benefit mandates at this time because if a state plans to include any services beyond the essential health benefits package that were not mandated prior to 2012, the state must defray the cost of the additional service through a payment to the enrollee or the plan.

In the lead-up to passage of the ACA, there was significant debate about whether to allow or require plans to offer abortion and contraceptive services. In fact, the abortion debate was so divisive it almost doomed the entire health reform bill at the 11th hour. A compromise was reached with the intent of keeping the status quo regarding federal funding for abortion services (i.e., limit federal funding for abortion services to cases where the life of the pregnant woman is in danger or the pregnancy is a result of rape or incest). Under the compromise, states may enact a law that prohibits plans that participate in their state exchanges from providing abortion services.

The ACA also provides coverage, without any cost-sharing, for all FDA-approved contraception methods. While contraception is considered a preventive service under the EHB standard, it is not specifically listed in the statute (nor are other preventive services; instead the statute references guidelines such as the United States Preventive Services Task Force A and B recommendations). Contraceptive coverage is part of a separate provision that includes women's preventive services identified by the Health Resources and Services Administration. Because this guideline is created by an administrative agency, each successive administration has the power to change the list of approved women's preventive services without needing congressional approval. The Obama administration exempted certain entities from being required to provide contraception coverage due to religious objections.[75] The required breadth of this exemption is the subject of numerous lawsuits and remains unsettled at this time. The Trump administration is considering a new administrative rule that would significantly broaden the group of employers and insurers who would qualify for the exemption based on religious or moral grounds.[76]

Given the Trump administration's policies intended to restrict access to abortion services (e.g., supporting the defunding of Planned Parenthood) and contraceptive devices (e.g., by broadening the religious objection exemption), it is worth noting what actions states have taken on these issues. As of July 2017, 25 states have enacted laws that restrict abortion services in exchange plans, though only Tennessee and Louisiana prohibit all abortion coverage.[77] If a state does not enact such a law and a plan chooses to offer abortion services in other circumstances, the plan must create separate financial accounts to ensure that federal premium and cost-sharing subsidies are not used toward those abortion services. In addition, at least one of the multistate plans is required not to provide abortion services beyond those that are currently allowed with federal funding. As with most compromises, neither side was entirely pleased with the outcome. Those who want more restrictive abortion policies found the separate accounting process to be a meaningless exercise, whereas those who want more permissive abortion policies were disturbed by the ability of states to prohibit plans from offering abortion services. In terms of contraception, 28 states require insurers that cover prescription drugs to cover all FDA-approved contraception methods. Three states require contraception to be provided without cost-sharing. Twenty states provide some type of exemption from their mandate, while eight states do not allow employers or insurers to refuse to cover contraception.[78]

The ACA also created a "catastrophic coverage" option that must include EHBs.[79] A catastrophic plan may be offered only to individuals under the age of 30 who would be exempt from the individual mandate requirement due to hardship or affordability exemptions. These plans require coverage of EHBs, certain preventive services without cost-sharing, and at least three primary care visits each year before meeting the deductible.[79] Individuals may not use premium tax credits to subsidize catastrophic plans, which typically have low premiums but very high deductibles.

BOX 3 Discussion Questions

There was a lengthy debate about whether to include a public option in health reform. A public option is some type of government-run health plan that would be available to compete with private plans. A public option could exist within the health exchange model or outside of it. Instead of a public option, Congress voted to require the Office of Personnel Management, which runs the Federal Employees Health Benefit Program, to contract with at least two multistate plans in every state health insurance exchange.

What are the pros and cons of having a public option? Does the Office of Personnel Management compromise achieve all or some of the goals of having a public option? Why do you believe the Office of Personnel Management compromise was acceptable to legislators but the public option was not?

Premium and Cost-Sharing Subsidies

One key difference among the exchange plans is the cost to the enrollee. Four levels of plans may be offered, and they are distinguished by their actuarial value. Actuarial value is the average share of covered benefits generally paid by the insurer based on the cost-sharing provisions in the plan. The higher the actuarial value, the more the plan pays for a given set of services. For example, in a plan with 70% actuarial value, the plan pays 70% of the cost of services on average across all enrollees, while enrollees pay 30%. Actuarial value is set by average cost, but any single enrollee in that plan may pay more or less than 30% of the cost of services. In general, plans with a higher actuarial value will also have higher premiums to cover the cost of providing services to enrollees. A plan with lower premiums could have higher cost-sharing (copays or deductibles) to offset the lower premium. The four ACA-approved plan levels by actuarial value are bronze (60% actuarial value), silver (70% actuarial value), gold (80% actuarial value), and platinum (90% actuarial value). Plans must offer at least one silver-level and one gold-level option in each exchange in which they participate.

The ACA includes premium tax credits and cost-sharing subsidies to help make it affordable for people to purchase health insurance in a state exchange. Given the mandate to purchase insurance, it was necessary to include some assistance to make it possible for low-income individuals to comply with the new requirement. The tax credits and subsidies were available starting in 2014, the same year the individual mandate and the state health insurance exchanges went into effect. In 2017, 8.7 million people (84% of marketplace enrollees) received a premium tax credit, and 5.9 million people (57% of marketplace enrollees) receive a cost-sharing subsidy.[80]

Premium tax credits are available to individuals who are eligible to purchase health insurance in state exchanges, have incomes between 100% and 400% of the federal poverty level, are not eligible for Medicaid, CHIP, or Medicare, and do not have access to affordable employer-sponsored health insurance. (An employer plan is not considered affordable if it does not cover at least 60% of covered benefits or if the employee's share of premium contributions exceeds 9.5% of the employee's income.) In 2017, 400% of the poverty level was $48,240 for an individual and $98,400 for a family of four.[81] The tax credits are advanceable and refundable, meaning they are available when health insurance is purchased and regardless of whether the individual owes any taxes. Cost-sharing subsidies (i.e., federal funds provided to assist individuals with the purchase of insurance) are available to people who earn between 100% and 250% of the poverty level. Under the ACA, individuals with income less than 133% of the poverty level will be eligible for Medicaid beginning in 2014 in those states that elected to implement the ACA's Medicaid eligibility expansion.

The amount of the premium tax credit is tiered based on income and set so individuals will not have to pay more than a certain percentage of their income on premiums (**TABLE 2**). The tax credit amount is based on the cost of the second-lowest-cost silver plan in the exchange and location where the individual is eligible to purchase insurance. Individuals who want to purchase a more expensive plan have to pay the difference in cost between the second-lowest-cost silver plan and the plan they prefer to purchase. Under the ACA, HHS will adjust the premium people are expected to pay to reflect that premium costs typically grow faster than income levels.

TABLE 2 Premium Tax Credit Schedule	
Income Level by Federal Poverty Level (FPL)	**Premium as a Percentage of Income**
100%–133% FPL	2% of income
133%–150% FPL	3%–4% of income
150%–200% FPL	4%–6.3% of income
200%–250% FPL	6.3%–8.05% of income
250%–300% FPL	8.05%–9.5% of income
300%–400% FPL	9.5% of income

For example, assume Bob's income is 250% of poverty (about $31,000 for an individual), and the cost of the second-lowest-cost silver plan in Bob's area is $5,700. Under the premium tax credit schedule, Bob will pay no more than 8.05% of his income, or $2,495. Bob's tax credit is $3,205, which is $5,700 minus $2,495.[82]

Cost-sharing subsidies are available to help low-income people reduce the amount of out-of-pocket spending on health insurance (**TABLE 3**). The subsidies are tiered by income level and set so that plans pay a higher percentage of service costs. In other words, they are set to increase the actuarial value of the plan for low-income individuals.

In addition to the premium tax credits and cost-sharing subsidies, the ACA limits the overall amount of out-of-pocket costs paid by individuals with incomes up to 400% of poverty (**TABLE 4**). The limits are based on the maximum out-of-pocket costs for health savings accounts ($6,550 for single coverage, $13,100 for family coverage in 2017) and will be indexed annually.

TABLE 3 Cost-Sharing Subsidy Schedule	
Income Level by Federal Poverty Level (FPL)	**Actuarial Value**
100%–150% FPL	94%
150%–200% FPL	87%
200%–250% FPL	73%

TABLE 4 Out-of-Pocket Spending Limits	
Income Level by Federal Poverty Level (FPL)	**Out-of-Pocket Limit**
100%–200% FPL	2/3 of maximum
200%–300% FPL	1/2 of maximum
300%–400% FPL	1/3 of maximum

BOX 4 Discussion Questions

Premium and cost-sharing subsidies are estimated to cost $919 billion over the years 2018–2027. Is this a good use of resources? Are these subsidies well designed? Are they sufficient to make health insurance affordable? Do they cover people with incomes that are too high? Should they cover more people?

The insurance subsidies have been at the center of litigation and political maneuvering and are discussed later. These subsidies, and in turn, the viability of the ACA overall, were at risk due to a lawsuit that challenged the legality of subsidies provided to the millions of people in the states that use a federally operated insurance exchange instead of setting up a state-based exchange.[83] Congress wrote in the ACA that federal subsidies were available to individuals who purchased health insurance through exchanges that were "established by the State." As part of the law's implementation process, the Internal Revenue Service (IRS) issued a regulation indicating that federal subsidies were available to individuals who purchased health insurance in either state-run or federally operated exchanges.[84] The individuals who brought the lawsuit argued that the IRS regulation was unlawful because it contradicted the language of the ACA. In essence, the court case boiled down to the meaning of the four words "established by the State": When read contextually against the rest of the ACA, were federally operated exchanges included in exchanges "established by the State" or, were federal subsidies reserved only for individuals in states that established their own state-run exchange?

In a 6–3 decision in *King v. Burwell*, the U.S. Supreme Court upheld the ACA's statutory and regulatory scheme, allowing federal subsidies to flow to individuals who purchase insurance in both state-run and federally operated exchanges.[85] Instead of reading the four words in question in a vacuum, Chief Justice Roberts, writing for the majority, viewed the phrase "established by the State" in the context of the overall purpose of the law. Doing otherwise, according to the court, would bring about "the type of calamitous result [insurance market failure] that Congress plainly meant to avoid" in crafting the ACA in the first place. Noting that the court's duty is to construe statutes as a whole, not "isolated provisions," Chief Justice Roberts wrote: "Congress passed the Affordable Care Act to improve health insurance markets, not to destroy them. If at all possible, we must interpret the [ACA] in a way that is consistent with the former, and avoids the latter. [The IRS regulation] can fairly be read consistent with what we see as Congress's plan, and that is the reading we adopt."[85]

In upholding the subsidies, the court differed in its reasoning from some lower federal courts that nonetheless also upheld the subsidies across all exchanges. These lower courts found the ACA's subsidy language ambiguous and therefore deferred to the agency (the IRS) that was tasked with interpreting the statute. In a critical move, the Supreme Court instead ruled that because the availability of tax credits was an issue with "deep economic and political significance" to the country, the meaning of the subsidy language should be interpreted by the court itself, rather than left to agency discretion. This decision means that the only way the subsidy language can be altered in the future is through congressional action, rather than by a future president whose administration might reinterpret the language more narrowly. This makes it far more likely that the subsidies will remain available in all exchanges—regardless of whether a state or the federal government operates them—going forward.

In addition to saving insurance subsidies for millions of Americans, the decision in *King v. Burwell* could have additional ramifications. Taken in conjunction with *NFIB v. Sebelius* (the 2012 Supreme Court decision upholding the constitutionality of the ACA), lower courts may read *King*'s direction to interpret the ACA as a congressional effort to improve insurance markets as a signal to forestall future litigation against the law. Furthermore, in states that have had difficulty setting up or operating their own exchange, the decision may encourage them to rely on the federal exchange apparatus; because there is no longer the threat that insurance subsidies could be easily untethered from federally facilitated exchanges, the use of such an exchange could become relatively more attractive.

Employer Mandate

As written in the ACA, employers with 50 or more employees and at least 1 employee who qualifies for a tax credit were required to offer affordable health insurance or pay a penalty beginning in 2014. The Obama administration twice delayed implementation of the mandate to smooth the transition, but the mandate itself did not change. Under the mandate, covered employers have three options: (1) provide affordable health insurance and not pay a penalty, (2) provide health insurance not considered affordable and pay a penalty, or (3) do not provide health insurance and pay a penalty. The penalties are based on whether an employer offers health insurance and whether any full-time employees take a premium tax credit. The amount of the penalty increases over time based on the national increase in premium costs. The employer mandate was put in place to encourage employers to continue offering or start offering health insurance. Without such a mandate, employers may have found it profitable not to offer health insurance and let their employees purchase health insurance through state exchanges, shifting more of the costs of health reform to the public sector and taxpayers.

For employers that do not offer health insurance and have at least one full-time employee who takes the premium tax credit, the penalty is $2,000 per employee after the first 30 employees. In other words, if such an employer has 50 employees, the employer would pay a $40,000 penalty ($2,000 × 20 employees).

Employers that offer health insurance do not pay a penalty if the insurance is considered affordable. Insurance is affordable if the plan has an actuarial value of at least 60% or if the premiums do not cost more than 9.5% of an employee's income. Employees who would have to pay more than 9.5% of their income on premiums have the option to purchase insurance through an exchange and receive a premium tax credit.

Employers who provide unaffordable insurance have to pay a penalty for each employee who takes a tax credit, not counting the first 30 employees (the 30-employee exception was included in the law due to Congress's concern about the impact of the employer mandate on small businesses). The penalty is $3,000 per employee who takes a tax credit but may not exceed $2,000 times the number of employees over 30. For example, if the employer has 50 employees and offers unaffordable coverage, the employer would pay a maximum penalty of $40,000 ($2,000 × 20). If only 10 employees take a tax credit, the penalty would be $30,000 ($3,000 × 10). If all 50 employees take a tax credit, the penalty would be $40,000, which is the maximum penalty allowed, not $150,000 ($3,000 × 50).

Employers must offer vouchers to employees who earn up to 400% of poverty level, would have to pay premiums between 8% and 9.8% of their income, and choose to enroll in a state exchange. The voucher is equal to the amount the employer would have paid for the employee in the employer's plan and is used to offset premium costs in the exchange plan. Employees who receive vouchers are not eligible for subsidies.

Given their smaller pool of employees, small businesses have often found it quite expensive to offer health insurance to their employees. In addition to exempting businesses with fewer than 50 employees from the employer mandate (and creating a health insurance exchange for small businesses), Congress also included a small business tax credit to encourage these employers to provide coverage. Employers are eligible for the tax credit if they have fewer than 25 full-time-equivalent employees, average annual wages under $50,000, and pay for at least half of the cost of health insurance coverage for their employees. The tax credit covers a portion of the cost of the employer's contribution toward employees' premiums. The credit is capped based on the average premium costs in the employer's geographical area and phases out as firm size and annual wages increase.

Because the employer mandate will lead to increased costs for certain employers (as the result of either paying ACA penalties or providing new insurance coverage), some of these employers may be influenced to offset new costs by employing more part-time workers (at the expense of full-time employment) and/or capping the number of workers they hire at 49.[86] While several analyses indicate that the effects to the labor market of these concerns may in fact be modest,[86,87] the authors of one study[86] nonetheless go so far as to advocate for eliminating the employer mandate altogether. They argue that doing so would actually not reduce overall insurance coverage significantly, would eliminate any market distortions that could result from changes in employer hiring practices, and would have the added benefit of lessening employer opposition to the ACA.[86]

Changes to the Private Insurance Market

In addition to creating a new marketplace for private insurance through state exchanges, the ACA includes a variety of changes to private health insurance rules and requirements. These requirements cover everything from rate setting, to benefits, to who must be covered. Although the overall health reform law is controversial, many of these private market reforms have overwhelming support. Together, these changes filled in gaps left by the private market that many people believed were unfair to consumers.

The following coverage changes took effect in 2010:

- **Preexisting conditions:** Individual and group plans may not exclude children due to their health status or based on preexisting conditions.
- **Dependent coverage:** Individual and group plans must provide dependent coverage up to age 26.
- **Preventive services:** New health plans may not impose cost-sharing for certain preventive services, including the following:
  - Preventive services with an A or B rating from the U.S. Preventive Services Task Force
  - Immunizations recommended by the Centers for Disease Control and Prevention's Advisory Committee on Immunization Practice
  - Preventive care and screening for women based on guidelines to be issued by the Health Resources and Services Administration
- **Coverage limits:** Individual and group plans may not impose lifetime dollar limits on coverage (and the ability to impose annual limits on the dollar value of coverage is prohibited as of 2014).
- **Rescission:** Individual and group plans may not rescind coverage except in the case of fraud.
- **Appeals:** New health insurance plans must have an effective appeals process that includes an external review option.

Congress also focused on the issue of how insurers determine premium rates and what they spend those resources on within their plans. The ACA charges HHS with establishing an annual process to review "unreasonable" increases in premiums.[1(§1003)] As of 2016, 43 states and the District of Columbia had some type of rate review law in place for all of their insurance markets, and the federal process is intended to work with, not preempt, those state laws.[88] HHS issued the final rule on this subject in May 2011. In addition, the ACA requires that plans spend at least 85% (large-group plans) or 80% (small-group or individual plans) of their premium dollars on medical care and quality improvement services, not administrative or other expenses (e.g., profits). Regulations clarifying this medical loss ratio, as it is called, took effect on January 1, 2011.[89] Insurers must provide enrollees with a rebate if they do not spend the requisite percentage on clinical and quality improvement services.

A number of significant insurance changes took place in 2014 alongside implementation of the individual mandate and health insurance exchanges:

- **Guaranteed issue and renewability:** Individual and group plans may not exclude or charge more to individuals based on preexisting conditions or health status in the individual market, small-group market, and exchanges.
- **Rate variation limits:** Premium rates may only vary based on age, geographical area, family composition, and tobacco use in the individual market, small-group market, and exchanges.
- **Coverage limits:** Individual and group plans may not place annual dollar limits on coverage.
- **Essential health benefits:** Insurers providing coverage to small businesses, individuals, and in the exchanges have to provide essential health benefits

through one of four plan categories (bronze, silver, gold, or platinum) and adhere to annual cost-sharing limits.

■ **Wellness plans:** Employers may offer rewards that reduce the cost of coverage to employees for participating in a wellness plan.

These private market changes do not affect all plans equally. Plans in small-group or nongroup markets must follow these rules whether or not they are offered in an exchange. On the other hand, the ACA included two significant exceptions to these reforms. First, insurance plans that were in existence when the ACA was signed into law are referred to as "grandfathered plans" and are subject to some, but not all, of the new rules. The grandfathered plans must follow new requirements relating to preexisting conditions, lifetime and annual limits, waiting period limits, and dependent coverage rules. These plans are exempt, however, from having to provide essential health benefits, preventive services without copays, and limited cost-sharing, although many of the large employer plans already have some of these features.[90] A plan may retain its grandfathered status as long as it does not make significant changes to plan benefits or cost-sharing rules. If it loses its grandfathered status, the plan will have to meet all applicable requirements.[91] In 2016, just under one-quarter of all employers offered at least one grandfathered plan, and the same percentage of covered workers were enrolled in a grandfathered plan.[92]

The second major exception is for self-funded plans. These are plans where an employer does not buy insurance from a company but instead takes on the insurance risk itself. Self-funded plans are exempt from state law and subject to federal rules under ERISA. Self-funded plans must adhere to ACA rules regarding dependent coverage, cost-sharing for preventive services, annual and lifetime limits, and waiting period limits, but do not need to comply with essential health benefit requirements.[93]

Financing Health Reform

Congress financed health reform primarily through Medicare and Medicaid savings, excise taxes and fees on the healthcare industry, changes to the income tax code, a tax on some health insurance plans, and expected individual and employer payments for violating insurance mandates. Several of these financing changes were made as part of the deals the Obama administration struck with various stakeholders.

The ACA's main financing features are as follows:

■ **Medicare provider reimbursement:** Reduces "market basket" or cost updates for inpatient and outpatient hospital reimbursement. Reduces payments for preventable hospital readmissions and hospital-acquired infections. Includes productivity adjustments (an adjustment in the Medicare physician fee schedule pertaining to physician productivity) for certain providers that will result in lower reimbursement rates.

■ **Medicare Advantage payments:** Reduces reimbursement rates and imposes cost-sharing limits for Medicare's managed care plans.

■ **Medicare Part A (hospital insurance):** Increases Medicare Part A tax rate for high-income earners.

■ **Medicare premiums:** Reduces Medicare Part D (prescription drug) premium subsidy for high-income beneficiaries.

- **Medicare employer subsidy:** Eliminates tax deduction for employers who receive a Medicare Part D (prescription drug coverage) subsidy.
- **Disproportionate share hospital (DSH) payments:** Reduces Medicare payments to DSH hospitals. Payments may increase over time based on percentage of uninsured served and uncompensated care provided. Reduces Medicaid DSH payments and requires HHS to develop a new funding formula.
- **Medicaid prescription drugs:** Increases rebates that drug manufacturers give to state Medicaid programs
- **Income tax code provisions:** Increases the threshold from 7.5 to 10% of adjusted gross income to claim deduction for unreimbursed medical expenses. Prohibits purchasing over-the-counter drugs with tax-free savings accounts, increases the tax burden on distributions not used for qualified medical expenses, and limits the amount individuals may put in accounts toward medical expenses.
- **Health industry fees:** Imposes a 10% tax on indoor tanning services, 2.3% tax on all taxable medical devices, annual fees on the pharmaceutical manufacturing sector, and fees on the health insurance sector.
- **Health insurance plans:** Imposes a tax on employer-sponsored health insurance plans with aggregate expenses that exceed $10,200 for individual coverage or $27,500 for family coverage.

Although it is the responsibility of the CBO to estimate the cost of legislation as it is written, time-bound cost estimates (e.g., a 10-year estimate) have their limitations. First, the CBO must assume that all the provisions in the bill will be implemented as written. One of the most unpopular cost-saving tools—a tax on more generous health insurance plans—is not slated to take effect until 2018. Second, because the 10-year estimate, by design, does not consider costs beyond the first decade, some expected costs are not included in the estimate. Third, different

BOX 5 Discussion Questions

The ACA includes a tax on insurers for more generous health plans. Because it is likely insurers will pass on the cost of the tax to consumers, the idea behind the tax is to provide incentives for people to choose lower-cost plans. In theory, the less money employers spend on healthcare costs (and other fringe benefits), the more they will spend on wages. The income tax paid for by workers on their higher wages will provide revenue that can be used to pay for health reform. In addition, people may be less likely to obtain unnecessary care if fewer services are covered by their plan or if cost-sharing is higher.

Is it likely that employers will trade lower benefits for higher wages? Are there times or industries where this trade-off is more or less likely to occur?

In 2016 the average cost of premiums for an employer plan was $6,435 for single coverage and $18,142 for family coverage.[92] Beginning in 2018, plans that exceed $10,200 for individual coverage and $27,500 for family coverage are taxed. Congress rejected lower thresholds for the tax ($8,500/$23,000) that would have raised an estimated $149 billion. Did Congress pick the right thresholds for the tax? Should they be higher or lower?

Why did Congress delay implementation of the tax until 2018? What are the pros and cons to having the tax start well after the main provisions of health reform are in place?

methodologies may be used to calculate costs. Fourth, cost estimates cannot account for provisions that are left out of a bill. For these reasons, cost estimates should not be taken as the final word on the cost of any bill, because changes in political will can undermine the best projections.

Public Health, Workforce, Prevention, and Quality

The ACA also includes a variety of programs and pilot projects that focus on improving quality of care and increasing access to preventive care. These provisions show both a commitment to these issues and the limitations of that commitment. For example, the Prevention and Public Health Fund was created to improve the nation's public health and is scheduled to provide $14 billion to support these activities from 2018 to 2027.[94] Congress, however, has the ability to redirect resources, and the prevention fund lost over $6 billion in 2012 when money intended for the fund was used to offset a scheduled reduction in Medicare physician payments, and it lost another $68 million in 2016 due to budget sequestration.[94,95] In addition, while task forces and pilot programs can be useful tools to try out new ideas and gather data to inform future changes, their temporary nature can also mean that progress ends once the experiment is over, especially in tight budget times. Whether these steps lead to lasting reform and needed change in the delivery of health care and in public health practice remains to be seen.

The ACA includes a wide range of quality improvement activities that fall into three main categories: evaluating new models of delivering health care, shifting reimbursement from volume to quality, and overall system improvement.[96] New models of healthcare delivery include Accountable Care Organizations, which combine a variety of providers who collectively assume responsibility for the cost and quality of patient care, and Patient-Centered Medical Homes, which provide comprehensive and coordinated primary care. Reimbursement reforms include strategies such as penalizing hospitals with high rates of hospital-acquired infections or providing bonuses or penalties based on performance on quality measurements. Finally, overall system improvement efforts are highlighted by the National Strategy for Quality Improvement and the Patient-Centered Outcomes Research Institute (PCORI). The priorities of the National Strategy for Quality Improvement include improving delivery of healthcare services, patient outcomes, and population health. PCORI, a comparative effectiveness institute, was created to consider the clinical effectiveness of medical treatments. The idea behind comparative effectiveness is to determine which procedures, devices, and pharmaceuticals provide the best value for a given outcome. The institute is designed to supply information to help providers, patients, and others make decisions; Congress has stipulated, however, that findings from the institute may not be construed as mandates or recommendations for payment, coverage, or treatment decisions.

The ACA also provides funds to promote public health, wellness, and a stable and high-quality healthcare workforce. In addition to the Public Health and Prevention Fund, the law calls for the creation of a new regular corps and ready reserve corps to assist when public health emergencies occur. Also, a variety of programs and incentives are in place to promote employer wellness programs. Finally, the workforce shortage is addressed through graduate medical education reforms that promote primary care training; increases in scholarships and loans to support primary care providers and workforce diversity; and education, training, and loan repayment programs to address the primary care nursing shortage.

BOX 6 Discussion Questions

There is a debate about the proper age at which to start regular mammogram screenings to detect breast cancer in women who do not have specific risk factors for the disease. As of 2009, the U.S. Preventive Services Task Force recommends waiting until age 50 to begin mammogram screening for breast cancer and further recommends that screening should occur every 2 years. It also, stated, however, that the final decision about the initial timing and frequency of breast cancer screening should be made by the patient and her physician. In making its recommendations, the Task Force found that physicians would need to screen 1,000 women to save 1 woman's life and concluded that earlier and/or more frequent screening was not worth the harm associated with false positives (anxiety, unnecessary biopsies, overtreatment). Other organizations disagree with the U.S. Preventive Services Task Force and conclude that the lifesaving effects of more routine mammogram screening outweigh the potential harm. Thus, the American Cancer Society recommends having routine annual mammograms from age 45–54 (or 40 if the patient so chooses) and then every 2 years thereafter. The American College of Obstetricians and Gynecologists recommends starting annual mammograms at age 40.

The idea of comparative effectiveness research is to provide information about the value of different tools. Once that information is available, however, who should make the decisions about whether to provide coverage and reimbursement for a particular good or service? Can one objectively assess the potential harms and benefits associated with mammograms or other services or medications? Should decisions be made solely by the patient and treating provider? Does it matter if decisions affect taxpayers (for example, if a patient is covered by a government program such as Medicare or the Veterans Administration)?

Sources: United States Preventive Services Taskforce. Breast cancer: Screening. https://www.uspreventiveservicestaskforce.org/Page/Document/UpdateSummaryFinal/breast-cancer-screening1. Published January 2016. Accessed July 26, 2017; American College of Obstetricians and Gynecologists. ACOG statement on breast cancer screening guidelines. https://www.acog.org/About-ACOG/News-Room/Statements/2016/ACOG-Statement-on-Breast-Cancer-Screening-Guidelines. Published January 11, 2016. Accessed July 26, 2017; American Cancer Society. American Cancer Society guidelines for the early detection of cancer. https://www.cancer.org/healthy/find-cancer-early/cancer-screening-guidelines/american-cancer-society-guidelines-for-the-early-detection-of-cancer.html. Accessed July 26, 2017.

The U.S. Supreme Court's Decision in the Case of *National Federation of Independent Business v. Sebelius*

In November 2011, in the first of what would be several ACA-related decisions, the U.S. Supreme Court agreed to decide four issues related to the legality of the ACA, two of which remain relevant for purposes of this text: (1) whether Congress had the power under the federal Constitution to enact the individual insurance coverage requirement and (2) whether it was unconstitutionally coercive for Congress, through the ACA, to threaten to take away existing federal Medicaid funding from states that did not want to implement the Medicaid expansion.

In June of the following year, the court handed down a remarkable 5–4 decision in the case of *National Federation of Independent Businesses, et al. v. Sebelius, Secretary of Health and Human Services, et al.*[97] The opinion was surprising for two reasons: it defied expectation—few people thought that the entirety of the ACA would be found constitutional by a majority of the court—and because Chief Justice Roberts, a conservative, ended up in the majority with the court's relatively liberal members (Justices Ginsburg, Breyer, Sotomayor, and Kagan).

The court first tackled the question of whether Congress exceeded its authority in effectively forcing most everyone to carry health insurance. It concluded, not totally unexpectedly given the outcome of the court's more recent Commerce Clause decisions,[98] that the "individual mandate" amounted to an unconstitutional reach on the part of federal legislators:

> The individual mandate . . . does not regulate existing commercial activity. It instead compels individuals to become active in commerce by purchasing a product, on the ground that their failure to do so affects interstate commerce. Construing the commerce clause to permit congress to regulate individuals precisely because they are doing nothing would open a new and potentially vast domain to congressional authority.[97(p2587)]

Surprisingly, however, the court's analysis of the constitutionality of the individual mandate did not end there. The court majority pivoted to Congress's power to tax, and ruled that under this separate power, the individual mandate passed constitutional muster. The court wrote:

> The exaction the Affordable Care Act imposes on those without health insurance [i.e., the financial penalty assessed on those who do not obtain minimum health insurance coverage] looks like a tax in many respects. . . . In distinguishing penalties from taxes, this Court has explained that "if the concept of penalty means anything, it means punishment for an unlawful actor omission." While the individual mandate clearly aims to induce the purchase of health insurance, it need not be read to declare that failing to do so is unlawful. Neither the Act nor any other law attaches negative legal consequences to not buying health insurance, beyond requiring a payment to the IRS.[97(p2595)]

Read together, the Supreme Court's analysis of the individual mandate under the Commerce Clause and the Taxing and Spending Clause leads to the following conclusion: Although Congress could not outright *command* Americans to buy health insurance, it could *tax* those who chose not to.

Next, the court turned its attention to whether the ACA's Medicaid expansion was structured in a way that effectively, and unlawfully, coerced states into adopting it. Fully half of the states in the country—the 26 that sued to halt implementation of the ACA—believed the answer to be "yes." As originally passed into law, the ACA allowed the secretary of HHS to terminate *all* of a state's Medicaid funding in the event that the state failed to implement the Medicaid expansion—even those Medicaid funds that a state would receive that were unconnected to the expansion. This, the states argued, amounted to a coercively unacceptable choice: either adopt the ACA Medicaid expansion or potentially receive no federal Medicaid financing at all. As a result, they asked the court to rule that the Medicaid expansion itself was unconstitutional.

The court responded to this argument in two ways. On the one hand, it determined that the Medicaid expansion itself was perfectly constitutional; on the other hand, the court ruled that it was indeed unconstitutional for HHS to penalize states that did not adopt the expansion by terminating all Medicaid funding:

> The Constitution simply does not give Congress the authority to require the States to regulate. That is true whether Congress directly commands a State to regulate or indirectly coerces a State to adopt a federal regulatory system as its own.... When, for example, such conditions take the form of threats to terminate other significant independent grants, the conditions are properly viewed as a means of pressuring the States to accept policy changes.... Nothing in our opinion precludes Congress from offering funds under the Affordable Care Act to expand the availability of healthcare, and requiring that States accepting such funds comply with the conditions on their use. What Congress is not free to do is to penalize States that choose not to participate in that new program by taking away their existing Medicaid funding.[97(pp2602–2607)]

This twin ruling had the effect of making the ACA Medicaid expansion optional rather than mandatory, and states have been deciding individually whether to implement it. As of the time of this writing, 31 states and the District of Columbia have adopted the ACA's Medicaid expansion, while 19 states have not adopted the expansion (though note that the latter number is noticeably lower than the number of states (26) that originally argued in *NFIB v. Sebelius* that the Medicaid expansion was unconstitutionally coercive).[99]

States and Health Reform

Before the ACA and in the wake of numerous failed attempts at national health reform, states had been active players in health reform. Filling the gap left by the lack of federal action, states took steps to experiment with individual mandates, employer mandates, small business pools, and programs to reduce the number of uninsured. Although the ACA is a federal law, it is full of state obligations and opportunities for state innovation. Even though governors in many states have expressed opposition to health reform, many states will expend significant efforts toward implementing the ACA over the next several years. The implementation challenges facing states are compounded by the poor economy that has forced many to cut government agency personnel and budgets. States will have their hands full developing and running health insurance exchanges, regulating the private health insurance market, and implementing Medicaid changes.

The Supreme Court's decision to transform the ACA's Medicaid expansion from a mandatory program change to a state option has significant ramifications. As noted previously, 31 states and the District of Columbia have chosen to expand their Medicaid program under the ACA.[99] As a result, by February 2017 there were 16 million more enrollees than prior to the ACA, with most new enrollment occurring in expansion states.[100] The number of new Medicaid beneficiaries will ultimately depend on how many states eventually choose to expand their Medicaid program.

The court's decision drastically changed the blueprint of health reform. The ACA was designed assuming Medicaid expansion in every state, meaning that there would be uniform coverage across the country for individuals earning below 138% of the federal poverty level. Under this plan, Medicaid would provide insurance for the lowest-income individuals, while state exchanges (with the assistance of federal subsidies) and employer-sponsored insurance would provide coverage for those who had higher earnings. It is now estimated that in states that do not expand their Medicaid program, 2.5 million people with incomes below the poverty line will remain uninsured because their incomes are too high to qualify for the state's traditional Medicaid program, yet too low to be able to afford private insurance in the exchanges because they do not qualify for subsidies (because it was assumed Medicaid would be expanded nationally, premium subsidies are only available for individuals earning at least 100% of poverty).[101]

▶ Key Issues Going Forward

At the time of this writing, the Republican effort to repeal and replace the ACA has stalled. Many in the party want to keep working toward that goal while others, including the Senate leadership, appear ready to focus on other matters such as tax reform and passing a budget. Complicating matters further, President Trump is urging Republicans to keeping working on health reform, making it difficult to discern which issues—and which branch of government—will triumph in the coming year. Will Congress significantly change or dismantle the ACA, or will it move on to other policy debates? Will the Trump administration undermine the ACA through executive actions in the absence of congressional activity? Will continuing implementation concerns and market forces loom large? And what will be the political fallout, if any, from whatever does or does not happen to the ACA in this Congress? In the end, Congress may not make significant changes to the ACA, and as time passes, the law may become an accepted and welcome part of the fabric that holds together our healthcare and public health systems. Until that time comes to pass, however, we discuss here a few major political and implementation issues that will likely dominate the health reform discussion in the near term.

1. Congressional Activity

The Republicans gained control of both chambers of Congress and of the White House in the 2016 election. After 7 years of campaigning on (and winning with) a platform that included repealing and replacing the ACA, Republican legislators feel a strong obligation to keep their promise. While the party is unified in its opposition to the ACA, it has been less successful agreeing on a replacement plan. With a slim majority in the Senate (52 Republicans, 48 Democrats) and no Democrats supporting this effort, Republicans are finding it difficult to meet the demands of moderate Republicans who want to protect the ACA's insurance gains and conservative Republicans who want to eliminate as many ACA requirements, regulations, and taxes as possible. Republicans face a similar dilemma in the House, although they have a little more room for disagreement, because they can survive with 21 Republican defectors and still pass a bill without support from the Democrats.

Congress spent the better part of the spring and summer in 2017 wrestling with repeal and replacement bills. After much political drama, the House passed their replacement bill, the American Health Care Act of 2017 (AHCA), on May 4, 2017 by a narrow 217–213 margin.[102] Every Democrat and 20 Republicans voted against the bill. In the Senate, Republicans drafted their bill, the Better Care Reconciliation Act of 2017 (BCRA), which followed the same general contours of the AHCA. After barely mustering sufficient support to proceed with debate on the bill, the Senate voted against BCRA on July 25, 2017. All Democrats and nine Republicans opposed the bill.[103] The next day, all Democrats and seven Republicans also voted against a bill that would have simply repealed the ACA (effective in 2 years) and did not include any type of replacement.[104] This repeal-only bill actually passed Congress while President Obama was in office, but because members of Congress who voted for repeal knew that Obama would veto the bill, it was considered a protest vote more than an agreement on a policy position.

During the 2017 Senate debate, Sen. John McCain (R-AZ), who at the time had been recently diagnosed with aggressive brain cancer, provided a moment of high drama. His "no" vote was the third Republican vote (along with Sens. Lisa Murkowski (R-AL) and Susan Collins (R-ME)) that ultimately doomed what was referred to as the "skinny repeal" option.[105] The skinny repeal option eliminated just the individual and employer mandates as well as a tax on medical devices. It was a bill that few actually wanted to become law, and it was projected to increase premiums and drastically reduce the number of insured individuals. Even the senators who voted for the bill did so only after assurances that the House would not pass it. Why, then, move forward with a bill few supported? The goal was to reach a "conference committee" wherein the House and Senate could work to reach a repeal and replace compromise, which would then be sent back to each chamber for approval. At that point, the political pressure to support a compromise bill would have been immense. The vote for the skinny repeal bill was a vote to keep the health reform debate alive, but risked a result that few desired. In voting against this strategy, the three Republican senators who voted "no" urged their colleagues to move forward in a bipartisan manner and to follow regular order in the Senate (holding hearings, passing bills through committee, etc.)

Even though the primary legislative bills—the AHCA and BCRA—did not have sufficient support across Congress to become law, and some of their provisions may not have been allowed under reconciliation rules, it is worth considering the main features of the bills to understand the type of health reform changes many Republicans support (see **TABLE 5**). Overall, these bills reduced taxes, eliminated government mandates, lowered federal government spending, lowered premiums for some people while increasing them for others, phased out the Medicaid expansion under the ACA, and ended Medicaid as an entitlement program. According to the nonpartisan CBO, the effect of the bills would be to significantly increase the number of uninsured, significantly reduce the deficit, lower costs for young and healthy consumers, and increase costs for older and poorer consumers.[52,106]

Major industry players and a clear majority of the public opposed the proposed bills to repeal and replace the ACA. Industry groups such as hospitals, physicians, safety net providers, and insurers were concerned about the health and financial effects of the bills, while key conservative groups (e.g., Heritage Foundation, Club for Growth) did not think the bills made sufficient changes.[107] While 64% of respondents indicated either a preference to keep the ACA as it is or to modify it, a clear partisan divide existed.[108] Nine out of 10 Democrats supported keeping or modifying the ACA, while only 3 out of 10 Republicans agreed. Most Republicans (about 75%) indicated they wanted the ACA repealed and replaced at some point.[11] For these reasons, it is not surprising that many Republican legislators feared the ramifications of disappointing their conservative base and donors by not repealing the ACA more than they feared whatever hazards awaited if they supported a bill that was unpopular with their constituencies.

One thing Congress has not tried yet is a bipartisan approach. A clear majority of the public (71%) strongly prefers for Republicans and Democrats to work together on health reform, and a number of legislators from both sides of the aisle have indicated a desire to do so. While a partisan divide remains here as well, 41% of all Republicans and 46% of Trump supporters would like to see the parties work together.[108] After the failed Senate efforts, Sen. Lamar Alexander (R-TN), Chair of the Senate committee on Health, Education, Labor and Pensions, agreed to open bipartisan hearings on fixing the individual marketplace.[109] In addition, a group of bipartisan legislators from the House announced a plan to improve the ACA. Their

TABLE 5 Comparison of U.S. House and Senate ACA Replacement Bills

	AHCA (House)	**BCRA (Senate)**
Premium tax credits	Replaces with tax credits based on age only, not income or geographic area	Keeps tax credits, eligibility lowered to 350%, includes those under 100% FPL, tied to less expensive benchmark, change individual contribution levels so older consumers pay more
Individual mandate	Eliminates penalties; replace with 1 year 30% premium surcharge if lapse in coverage	Eliminates penalties, replaces with 6 month waiting period if lapse in coverage
Employer mandate	Eliminates penalties	Eliminates penalties
Medicaid expansion	Phases out at end of 2019	Phases out by end of 2024
ACA taxes	Eliminates most key taxes	Eliminates many key taxes, keeps Medicare surtax and investment tax on high-income earners
Essential health benefits	Allows state waivers to redefine	Allows state waivers to redefine
Medicaid program	Changes to block grant or per capita allotment in 2020; allows work requirements	Changes to block grant or per capita allotment in 2020; allows work requirements
Cost-sharing subsidy funds	Funds through 2019, repeals in 2020	Funds through 2019, repeals in 2020

(continues)

TABLE 5 Comparison of U.S. House and Senate ACA Replacement Bills *(continued)*

	AHCA (House)	BCRA (Senate)
Women's health services	Defunds Planned Parenthood for 1 year; redefines qualified plan to exclude plans that provide abortion services except for rape, incest, or life of mother in danger	Defunds Planned Parenthood for 1 year; redefines qualified plan tc exclude plans that provide abortion services except for rape, incest, or life of mother in danger
Private market rules	Keep guaranteed issue, dependent coverage until 26; preexisting condition protection remains	Keep guaranteed issue, dependent coverage until 26; preexisting condition protection remains; permits sale of noncompliant plans as long as selling one ACA-compliant plan
State stabilization pool	Provides $123 billion over 9 years	Provides $182 billion over 9 years
Public health prevention fund	Eliminates	Eliminates
Age rating band	Changes to 5-to-1 but allows for state variation	Changes to 5-to-1 but allows for state variation
CBO estimate— uninsured	23 million more uninsured by 2026	22 million more uninsured by 2026
CBO estimate— federal savings	$119 billion	$321 billion

strategy includes: paying low-income cost-sharing subsidies to insurers, providing federal funds to the states to create reinsurance funds and other programs to lower premiums, applying the employer mandate to employers with 500 (instead of 50) or more employees, redefining full-time employee as those who work 40 hours per week, obtaining clarification from HHS about a §1332 waiver process, and repealing the medical device tax.[110] They also recommend offsetting the federal funds spent on these ideas, but do not indicate how current funding should be cut.

The political difficulty of repealing and replacing the ACA is not surprising. It is always difficult to take away benefits once people have started to use them. Supporting a bill that would result in over 20 million people losing insurance is clearly more politically perilous than not supporting legislation (i.e., the ACA) that would deliver health insurance to 20 million people for the first time. This is particularly true for federal legislators who hail from states that (a) implemented the ACA's Medicaid expansion and (b) have Republican governors. Why? Much of the savings from the House and Senate bills came from reduced Medicaid spending, both through the elimination of the expansion and by changing the entire program from an entitlement program to a block grant or per capita allotment. In turn, states would either have had to absorb the federal spending reductions in their own budgets or absorb the healthcare costs of having more uninsured residents. Indeed, the proposed changes to Medicaid, which went well beyond repealing and replacing the ACA, resulted in many of the biggest criticisms from moderate Republicans. Also, Medicaid has become even more important to the nation now that it is grappling with an opioid epidemic, because Medicaid and CHIP cover approximately one-third of individuals with an opioid addiction. This is nearly double the share covered by Medicaid in 2005 and the increase is mostly due to the ACA Medicaid expansion.[111]

The Senate Republican leadership also made a difficult political situation even harder by alienating several of their own members when the leadership decided that the ACA repeal bills would be drafted in relative secret, ignored regular process (by not holding hearings, debates, mark-ups), used reconciliation to avoid a filibuster, and expected their members to vote on bills they had little time to review. Sen. John Cornyn (R-TX), the second-ranking Republican in the Senate, went so far as to say that knowing prior to the start of debate which bill the Republicans would be voting on was "a luxury we don't have."[112] This was a hard pill to swallow for many Republicans who vilified the Democrats for their partisan approach to passing the ACA and who mocked then-House Speaker Nancy Pelosi (D-CA) for saying, "we have to pass the healthcare bill so that you can find out what's in it."[113] While ultimately Republican leaders were not successful in getting the legislation passed, they decided that the negative ramifications of these hardball tactics were easier to survive than the negative publicity of a drawn-out process where opposition groups could mobilize their resources.

2. The Trump Administration

Even if Congress cannot agree on a new health reform bill, the Trump administration wields significant power over the future of health reform through its executive authority. The key question is whether President Trump will follow through on his threat to "let Obamacare fail" with the goal of (a) pinning the collapse on Democrats and (b) forcing Democrats to negotiate with Republicans on a repeal and replacement bill.[114] Trump has asserted that "Republicans are not going to own [Obamacare's collapse]," but because Republicans hold power in Congress and the White House, they may end up being blamed for future healthcare woes.[114]

So far, Trump's actions and indecision on health reform issues have negatively affected the ACA. On his first day in office, Trump signed an Executive Order that allowed HHS and other agencies to "exercise all authority and discretion available to them to waive, defer, grant exemptions from, or delay the implementation of any provision or requirement of the [ACA] that would impose a fiscal burden" on the states, individuals, or other entities involved in health care.[115] While the specific changes that could take place under this Order are unclear, the intent to free individuals and states from ACA obligations is unmistakable. The administration also proposed a rule to make it more difficult to sign up for insurance during a special enrollment period, shortened the length of the next open enrollment period, and made it easier for insurers to collect back premiums.[116,117] In addition, the administration weakened enforcement of the individual mandate by ordering the IRS to continue processing tax returns even if filers do not indicate whether they had insurance coverage.[116] Examples of other actions the administration could take include withdrawing the appeal of a lawsuit that could eliminate cost-sharing subsidies (discussed more later), granting more hardship waivers to exempt people from complying with the individual mandate, limiting advertising and outreach during the next open enrollment period, granting waivers to the states to allow Medicaid-related work requirements or increased cost-sharing, rewriting regulations to allow for skimpier benefits under the essential health benefits requirement, and eliminating contraceptives from the list of women's preventive services.[118,119,120]

3. Insurance Plan Premium Rates

One of the key issues to monitor going forward is the affordability of health insurance plans under the ACA. Most people were pleasantly surprised by premium rates for 2014 and 2015, although there was a lot of variation across the country. Insurers had incentive to keep premiums low because they wanted to encourage people to enroll in their health plans. In addition, there was limited information about who would be in the insurance pools that could have assisted insurers with premium rate setting, and many plans contracted with a narrower set of providers as a way to keep premiums low. After moving past the initial enrollment period, will insurance companies hike premiums in future years?

Going into 2018, insurers are facing significant uncertainty due to the political landscape. With Congress reviewing a variety of repeal and replacement plans and the Trump administration threatening to let ACA reforms fail, insurers do not know what to expect in the upcoming year, and uncertainty is not something that makes for a stable health insurance market. As a result, insurers are asking for delays in submitting premium rates, and some are even submitting two rates depending on the outcome of certain political decisions.[121] Many insurers that are submitting rates are asking for double digit increases (a review of silver plans in 8 states showed an average increase of 18%[122]), while other rate requests are even higher. For example, insurers in Maryland are asking for rate increases ranging from 18 to 60%, and in Connecticut the range is 15 to 34%. Nevada is requesting an average rate hike of 38%, and Colorado's request is similar, with an average increase of 41%.[123,124]

The main sources of uncertainty are whether the Trump administration will fund cost-sharing subsidies and enforce the individual mandate.[123] Cost-sharing subsidies offset the cost of care for low-income consumers. These subsidies have been the subject of litigation brought by House Republicans under the Obama administration (Originally *House v. Burwell*, now *House v. Price*). The lower court agreed with the plaintiffs' claim that the subsidies should not be funded because Congress did not appropriate money for that purpose. The Obama administration appealed. The Trump administration has not decided whether it will continue to appeal the case or support funding of the cost-sharing subsidies. Meanwhile, insurers do not know whether to expect the $7 billion owed to them for providing the subsidies in 2017 or the billions that would be owed to them in future years. In addition, other actions, such as not enforcing the individual mandate and limiting outreach efforts, make it less likely that healthier individuals will enroll in the plans, resulting in a sicker and more expensive pool.

One actuarial firm estimated that two-thirds of the rate hikes were based on these unknowns.[122] In addition, not paying the cost-sharing subsidies would actually increase federal spending by approximately $2 billion because higher premiums would result in higher-cost premium tax credits.[125] Even so, it is important to note there are other reasons that premiums are rising. These include: lower than expected enrollment, a sicker than anticipated pool, and the need to cover the ACA tax on health insurers.[126]

Some insurers are responding to the uncertainty by exiting the market, while other insurers have increased their offerings.[125] While thousands of enrollees were expected to be in counties in which no insurer is offering a product on their exchange in 2018 (referred to as "bare" counties), there are no longer any bare counties due to recent decisions by insurers (with prodding by state insurance agencies).[127] Given the rising premiums and reduced insurance offerings, there is a debate about whether the exchanges are collapsing or stabilizing. While some analyses show a stabilizing market, continued subsidy support and increased enrollment of healthier individuals are key factors to the long-term success of the exchanges.[128,129,130]

4. ACA Litigation

Legal challenges to the ACA did not end with the Supreme Court's *NFIB v. Sebelius* decision in 2012, and the Supreme Court has handed down rulings in other ACA lawsuits. In 2014 the court decided *Burwell v. Hobby Lobby*, which answered whether, under a federal statute called the Religious Freedom Restoration Act (RFRA), closely held private corporations have a legal right to refuse to comply with provisions of the ACA that require them to provide certain contraceptive coverage to employees. (A closely held corporation is one that has a limited number of shareholders; in the *Hobby Lobby* case, the plaintiffs were two private, for-profit companies owned by members of a single family—Hobby Lobby Stores [owned by Evangelical Christians] and Conestoga Wood Specialties [owned by Mennonites]). In a 5–4 decision, the court majority determined that the ACA's contraception mandate imposed a significant enough burden on the plaintiff companies' exercise of their beliefs so as to violate RFRA. Then in 2015, the Supreme Court decided *King v. Burwell*, which, as described earlier, held that subsidies available under the ACA to help individuals and small businesses buy insurance were available whether the insurance was purchased through a state-run or federally facilitated insurance exchange. Most recently, in 2016, the Court heard *Zubik v. Burwell*, a case that is an offshoot of its earlier decision in *Burwell v. Hobby Lobby*. After the *Hobby Lobby* decision, the Obama Administration offered an accommodation to religious entities that objected to the requirement to provide contraceptive coverage without cost-sharing: simply inform HHS of your objection and identify your insurer, at which point HHS would take responsibility for ensuring that contraceptive services are provided by the insurer without the involvement of the religious organization. The accommodation, however, was not acceptable to a number of religious entities, which filed their own RFRA lawsuits. Over time, nine federal appellate courts ruled that the accommodation did not substantially burden the entities' exercise of religion; however, one appellate court ruled the opposite way, creating a division that the Supreme Court wanted to clear up. Eventually, the Supreme Court—likely split four-to-four on the merits by this time (i.e., after Justice Scalia died and the Senate failed to hold hearings on his replacement) and hoping to spark a compromise among the litigants— remanded the cases to the lower courts without a definitive answer.

At the time of this writing, all but one of these remanded cases remain pending in the appellate courts. In August 2017, the Third Circuit Court of Appeals ruled by a 2–1 margin in favor of the federal government in *Real Alternatives v. HHS*. Specifically, the two judges in the majority ruled that (1) the government need not exempt from the mandatory coverage requirement an employer that objects on moral, as opposed to religious, grounds; and (2) individuals who object to contraceptives on religious grounds need not be allowed to purchase insurance that does not cover contraceptives.

In addition to *Zubik v. Burwell* and *House v. Price* (the subsidies cost-sharing case described previously in the insurance premium section), there are two other types of cases bouncing around the federal courts that are worth noting. The first type is a set of cases (nearly two dozen in all) that involves the ACA's risk corridor program, which was intended to compensate insurers who ended up with costlier risk pools than other insurers. Two of these cases have recently reached the Federal Circuit Court of Appeals: *Land of Lincoln Mutual Health Insurance Co. v. United States* and *Moda Health Plan, Inc. v. United States*. In these cases, insurers claim that the federal government must pay the full amount owed under the risk corridor formula, rather than just a *pro rata* share of the funds collected under the program.

The second type is a single case, *Franciscan Alliance v. Burwell*, brought by several religious organizations and some states. It challenges a regulation promulgated under ACA section 1557, which prohibits discrimination on the basis of race, color, national origin, sex, age, or disability in certain health programs or activities. The challenged regulation, which specifically prohibits discrimination on the basis of gender identity or termination of pregnancy, was originally placed under a nationwide preliminary injunction (meaning that at the moment, the rule cannot be enforced) in December 2016 by a federal judge in Texas. The judge determined that the regulation's prohibition against sex discrimination based on gender identity was impermissible because, according to him, the term "sex" as used in the ACA refers to biological and anatomical differences between males and females as determined at birth. An appeal to the Fifth Circuit Court of Appeals is pending.

Given these and other lawsuits still to come, it is unlikely that the Supreme Court has cleared the ACA from its docket. However, irrespective of whether the Supreme Court hands down ACA-related cases in the future, what bears keeping in mind is that judicial decisions may continue to shape the contours of the ACA for years to come.

▶ Conclusion

After decades of trying and against the predictions of numerous experts, the United States passed a health reform law that provides insurance coverage on a more universal scale than ever before, includes protections for individuals who have been historically excluded from the insurance market, and shows a concern for improving healthcare quality and access to preventive care. From a philosophical perspective, the ACA moves America toward a society where (almost) everyone is expected to have adequate access to affordable health insurance.

Under this perspective, health insurance is considered both an obligation and a right: individuals are required to obtain insurance and the government is obligated to make it affordable and accessible. At the same time, there remains in some quarters strong philosophical and political opposition to the ACA, which continues to be challenged both legislatively and in the courts. Because of this opposition and because the ACA is still not close to engendering the type of support reserved for, say, Medicare, the full story of the ACA is far from being completed.

▶ References

1. Patient Protection and Affordable Care Act, Pub. L. No. 111–148.
2. Gordon C. *Dead on Arrival: The Politics of Health Care in Twentieth-Century America*. Princeton, NJ: Princeton University Press; 2003.
3. Blake CH, Adolino JR. The Enactment of National Health Insurance: A Boolean Analysis of Twenty Advanced Industrial Countries. *J Health Politics Policy Law*. 2001;26:670–708.
4. Jost TS. Why Can't We Do What They Do? National Health Reform Abroad. *J Law Med Ethics*. 2004;32:433–441.
5. Kaiser Family Foundation. *Kaiser health tracking poll: election 2008*. http://kff.org/health-reform /poll-finding/toplines-kaiser-health-tracking-poll-election-2008-3/. Published October 20, 2008. Accessed August 2, 2017.
6. Kaiser Family Foundation. *Chartpack: Kaiser health tracking poll: August 2009*. http://www .kff.org/health-costs/poll-finding/chartpack-kaiser-health-tracking-poll-august-2009/. Published August 1, 2009. Accessed August 2, 2017.
7. Pew Research Center. *Public support for single payer health coverage grows, driven by Democrats*. http://www.pewresearch.org/fact-tank/2017/06/23/public-support-for-single-payer-health -coverage-grows-driven-by-democrats/. Published June 23, 2017. Accessed July 18, 2017.
8. Newport F. U.S. still split on whether gov't should ensure healthcare. *Gallup*. http://www .gallup.com/poll/144839/Split-Whether-Gov-Ensure-Healthcare.aspx. Published November 18, 2010. Accessed August 2, 2017.
9. Steinhauer J. Old truths trip up G.O.P. on health law: A benefit is hard to retract. *New York Times*. https://www.nytimes.com/2017/07/17/us/politics/republican-party-health-care-law -obamacare.html. Published July 17, 2017. Accessed July 19, 2017.
10. Kaiser Family Foundation. *Kaiser health tracking poll—June 2017: ACA replacement plan, and Medicaid*. http://www.kff.org/health-reform/poll-finding/kaiser-health-tracking-poll-june -2017-aca-replacement-plan-and-medicaid/. Published June 23, 2017. Accessed July 18, 2017.
11. Kahn C, Erman M. Exclusive: Majority of Americans want Congress to move on from health reform—Reuters/Ipsos poll. *Reuters*. http://www.reuters.com/article/us-usa-healthcare-poll -idUSKBN1AE0RY. Published July 29, 2017. Accessed July 31, 2017.
12. Magness J. America's opposition to repealing Obamacare grows, particularly among Republicans. *McClatchy DC Bureau*. http://www.mcclatchydc.com/news/politics-government /article141562849.html. Published March 30, 2017. Accessed April 3, 2017.
13. Wynne B. Five lessons from the AHCA's demise. *Health Affairs Blog*. http://healthaffairs.org /blog/2017/03/27/five-lessons-from-the-ahcas-demise/. Published March 27, 2017. Accessed March 31, 2017.
14. Garrett TA. State balanced-budget and debt rules. *Economic Synopses*. https://files.stlouisfed. org/files/htdocs/publications/es/11/ES1133.pdf. Published October 19, 2011. Accessed July 19, 2017.)
15. Weissert CS, Weissert WG. *Governing Health: The Politics of Health Policy*. 2nd ed. Baltimore, MD: Johns Hopkins University Press; 2002.
16. Kondick K, Skelley G. Incumbent re-election rates higher than average in 2016. *Rasmussen Reports*. http://www.rasmussenreports.com/public_content/political_commentary/commentary_by_

kyle_kondik/incumbent_reelection_rates_higher_than_average_in_2016.PublishedDecember15, 2016. Accessed July 19, 2017.

17. Tax Policy Center Briefing Book. *What is reconciliation?* http://www.taxpolicycenter.org /briefing-book/what-reconciliation. Accessed July 19, 2017.

18. West DM, Heith D, Goodwin C. Harry and Louise Go to Washington: Political Advertising and Health Care Reform. *J Health Politics Policy Law.* 1996;21:35–68.

19. U.S. Bureau of the Census. *Income, poverty, and health insurance coverage in the United States: 2009.* Washington, DC: Bureau of the United States Census: 2010.

20. Feder J. Crowd-Out and the Politics of Health Reform. *J Law Med Ethics.* 2004;32:461–464.

21. Kaiser Family Foundation. *Chartpack: Kaiser health tracking poll—November 2009.* http://www .kff.org/kaiserpolls/upload/8019.pdf. Published November 1, 2009. Accessed August 8, 2017.

22. Starr P. *The Social Transformation of American Medicine: The Rise of a Sovereign Profession and the Making of a Vast Industry.* New York, NY: Basic Books; 1982.

23. National Archives and Records Administration. *Historical election results—electoral college box scores, 2000–2012.* http://www.recovery.gov/About/Pages/The_Act.aspx. Accessed June 29, 2015.

24. CNN. *Election center 2008.* http://www.cnn.com/ELECTION/2008/results/president/. Updated November 17, 2008. Accessed June 29, 2015.

25. Emergency Economic Stabilization Act of 2008, Pub. L. No. 110–343.

26. American Recovery and Reinvestment Act of 2009, Pub. L. No. 111–115.

27. Jones JM. Economy top issue for voters; size of gov't may be more pivotal. *Gallup.* http:// www.gallup.com/poll/144029/Economy-Top-Issue-Voters-Size-Gov-May%20-Pivotal.aspx. Published October 26, 2010. Accessed August 2, 2017.

28. Jones JM. Americans want next president to prioritize jobs, corruption. *Gallup.* http:// www.gallup.com/poll/156347/Americans-Next-President-Prioritize-Jobs%20-Corruption .aspx?utm_source=twitter&utm_medium=gallupnews&utm_campaign%20=syndication . Published July 30, 2012. Accessed August 2, 2017.

29. Obama talks about mother's cancer battle in ad. *CNN.* http://politicalticker.blogs.cnn .com/2007/09/21/obama-talks-about-mothers-cancer-battle-in-ad/. Published September 21, 2007. Accessed August 2, 2017.

30. Appleby J. health reform up in the air as the economy sinks. *USA Today.* https://usatoday30 .usatoday.com/news/health/2008-12-18-health_N.htm. Published December 20, 2008. Accessed August 2, 2017.

31. Obama's health care speech to Congress. *New York Times.* http://www.nytimes .com/2009/09/10/us/politics/10obama.text.html. Published September 9, 2009. Accessed August 2, 2017.

32. Kaiser Family Foundation. *Key findings: Kaiser health tracking poll—September 2009.* http:// www.kff.org/kaiserpolls/upload/7990.pdf. Published September 1, 2009. Accessed August 2, 2017.

33. Cohen J, Balz D. Opposition to Obama's health-reform plan is high, but easing. *Washington Post.* http://www.washingtonpost.com/wp-dyn/content/article/2009/09/13/AR2009091302962 .html\. Published September 14, 2009. Accessed August 2, 2017.

34. Condon S. Scott Brown win shakes up health care fight. *CBS News.* http://www.cbsnews.com /news/scott-brown-win-shakes-up-health-care-fight/. Published January 20, 2010. Accessed August 2, 2017.

35. Brown CB, O'Connor P. The fallout: Democrats rethinking health care bill. *Politico.* http:// www.politico.com/news/stories/0110/31693.html. Published January 21, 2010. Accessed August 2, 2017.

36. State of the Union: President Obama's speech. *ABC News.* http://abcnews.go.com/Politics%20 /State_of_the_Union/state-of-the-union–2010-president-obama-speech-transcript%20 /story?id=9678572&page=1. Published January 27, 2010. Accessed August 2, 2017.

37. Saad L. Obama and Bush: A contrast in popularity. *Gallup.* http://www.gallup.com /poll/111838/Obama-Bush-Contrast-Popularity.aspx. Published November 10, 2008. Accessed August 2, 2017.

38. Blumenthal D, Morone JA. *The Heart of Power: Health and Politics in the Oval Office.* Berkeley: University of California Press; 2009.

39. Morone J. Presidents and Health Reform: From Franklin D. Roosevelt to Barack Obama. *Health Aff.* 2010;29(6):1096–1100.

40. Oberlander J. Long Time Coming: Why Health Reform Finally Passed. *Health Aff.* 2010;29(6):1112–1116.

41. Kaiser Health News. *Letter from Obama to Sens Kennedy and Baucus.* June 3, 2009. http://khn.org/news/obamaletter/. Accessed August 2, 2017.

42. Affordable Health Care for America Act, H.R. 3962.

43. Patient Protection and Affordable Care Act, H.R. 3590.

44. Murray S, Kane P. Pelosi: House won't pass Senate bill to save health-care reform. *Washington Post.*http://www.washingtonpost.com/wp-dyn/content/article/2010/01/21/AR2010012101604.html. Published January 22, 2010. Accessed August 2, 2017.

45. Khan H. Health care bill aftermath: Rep. Patrick Kennedy hails dad's dream; Sen. John McCain sees heavy price. *ABC News.* http://abcnews.go.com/GMA/HealthCare/health-care-congress-passes-landmark-reform-obama-sign/story?id=10167139. Published March 22, 2010. Accessed August 2, 2017.

46. Graves JA, Nikpay SS. The changing dynamics of US health insurance and implications for the future of the Affordable Care Act. *Health Affairs.* 2017;36(2):297–305.

47. Health policy briefs: individual mandate. *Health Aff.* http://www.healthaffairs.org/healthpolicybriefs/brief.php?brief_id=14. Published January 13, 2010. Accessed August 2, 2017.

48. Agiesta J. CNN/ORC poll: public splits on revoking individual mandate. *CNN.* http://www.cnn.com/2017/03/07/politics/health-care-replacement-poll/index.html. Published March 7, 2017. Accessed July 23, 2017.

49. Burke, C. Rasmussen poll: most Americans oppose ACA's individual mandate. 46% oppose single-payer health care system. http://www.newsmax.com/Newsfront/Obamacare-majority-oppose-Rasmussen/2013/12/17/id/542447/. Published December 17, 2013. Accessed August 2, 2017.

50. Kaiser Family Foundation. *Kaiser health tracking poll: April 2014.* http://kff.org/health-reform/poll-finding/kaiser-health-tracking-poll-april-2014/. Published April 29 2014. Accessed August 2, 2017.

51. DiJulio B, Kirzinger A, Wu B, Brodie M. Data note: Americans' challenge with health care costs. *Kaiser Family Foundation.* http://www.kff.org/health-costs/poll-finding/data-note-americans-challenges-with-health-care-costs/. Published March 2, 2017. Accessed July 23, 2017.

52. Congressional Budget Office. *American Health Care Act—Cost Estimate.* https://www.cbo.gov/system/files/115th-congress-2017-2018/costestimate/americanhealthcareact.pdf. Published March 13, 2017. Accessed July 23, 2017.

53. Landler M, Shear MD. Enrollment exceeds Obama's target for health care act. *The New York Times.* http://www.nytimes.com/2014/04/18/us/obama-says-young-adults-push-health-care-enrollment-above-targets.html?_r=0. Published April 17, 2014. Accessed August 2, 2017.

54. Mills D. Young adults targeted in this fall's Obamacare enrollment drive. *Healthline.* Published June 29, 2016. Accessed July 23, 2017.

55. Mangan D. Obamacare young people sign ups nearly double. *CNBC.* http://www.cnbc.com/2015/12/22/obamacare-young-adult-sign-ups-nearly-double.html. Published December 2015. Accessed July 23, 2017.

56. U.S. Bureau of the Census. *Health insurance coverage in the United States: 2015.* Washington DC: Bureau of the United States Census; 2016.

57. 45 CFR, Parts 155 and 156.

58. Jost T. Implementing health reform: exemptions from the individual mandate. *Health Affairs Blog.* http://healthaffairs.org/blog/2013/06/27/implementing-health-reform-exemptions-from-the-individual-mandate/. Published June 27, 2013. Accessed August 2, 2017.

59. U.S. Const., art. I, §8.

60. *Heart of Atlanta Motel, Inc. v. United States*, 379 U.S. 241 (1964); *Wickard v. Filburn*, 317 U.S. 111 (1942); *Gonzales v. Raich*, 545 U.S. (2005).

61. Jost TS. State lawsuits won't succeed in overturning the individual mandate. *Health Aff.* 2010;29(6):1225–1228.

62. Shapiro I. State suits against health reform are well grounded in law—and pose serious challenges. *Health Aff.* 2010;29(6):1229–1233.

63. Kaiser Family Foundation. *Frequently asked questions: What is the health insurance marketplace?* http://kff.org/health-reform/faq/health-reform-frequently-asked-questions/. Accessed August 2, 2017.

64. Aron-Dine A. CBO correctly predicted historic gains under ACA. *Center on Budget and Policy Priorities.* https://www.cbpp.org/blog/cbo-correctly-predicted-historic-coverage-gains -under-aca. Published May 30, 2017. Accessed July 24, 2017.

65. Luhby T. What CBO got right—and wrong on Obamacare. *CNN Money.* http://money.cnn.com/2017/03/09/news/economy/cbo-obamacare/index.html. Published March 12, 2017. Accessed July 24, 2017.

66. Jost T. CMS announces plans to effectively end the SHOP exchange. *Health Affairs Blog.* http://healthaffairs.org/blog/2017/05/15/cms-announces-plans-to-effectively-end-the-shop -exchange/. Published May 15, 2017. Accessed July 24, 2017.

67. Centers for Medicaid and Medicare Services. *The future of the SHOP: CMS intends to allow small businesses using HealthCare.gov more flexibility when enrolling in healthcare coverage.* https://www.cms.gov/CCIIO/Resources/Regulations-and-Guidance/Downloads /The-Future-of-the-SHOP-CMS-Intends-to-Allow-Small-Businesses-in-SHOPs-Using -HealthCaregov-More-Flexibility-when-Enrolling-in-Healthcare-Coverage.pdf. Published May 15, 2017. Accessed July 24, 2017.

68. Congressional Budget Office. *Federal subsidies under the Affordable Care Act for health insurance coverage related to the expansion of Medicaid and nongroup health insurance: Tables from CBOs January 2017 baseline.* https://www.cbo.gov/sites/default/files /recurringdata/51298-2017-01-healthinsurance.pdf. Published January 2017. Accessed July 24, 2017.

69. Jost T. CBO lowers marketplace enrollment projections, increases Medicaid growth projections (updated). *Health Affairs Blog.* http://healthaffairs.org/blog/2016/01/26/cbo -lowers-marketplace-enrollment-projections-increases-medicaid-growth-projections/. Published January 26, 2016. Accessed July 24, 2017.

70. Kaiser Family Foundation. *Explaining health care reform: Questions about health insurance subsidies.* http://kff.org/health-reform/issue-brief/explaining-health-care-reform-questions -about-health/. Accessed August 7, 2017.

71. Kaiser Family Foundation. *State health insurance marketplace types, 2017.* http://www.kff .org/health-reform/state-indicator/state-health-insurance-marketplace-types/?currentTim eframe=0&sortModel=%7B%22colId%22:%22Location%22,%22sort%22:%22asc%22%7D. Accessed July 24, 2017.

72. Giovanelli J, Lucia KW, Corlette S. Implementing the Affordable Care Act: Revisiting the ACA's essential health benefits requirements. *The Commonwealth Fund.* http://www.commonwealthfund. org/~/media/files/publications/issue-brief/2014/oct/1783_giovannelli_implementing_aca_ essential_hlt_benefits_rb.pdf. Published October 2014. Accessed August 7, 2017.

73. Rosenbaum S, Teitelbaum J, Hayes K. Crossing the Rubicon: the impact of the Affordable Care Act on the content of insurance coverage for persons with disabilities. *Notre Dame J Law Ethics Public Policy.* 2011;25(2):527–562.

74. Giovanni J, Volk J, Lucia K, Williams A, Connor K. States revisit insurer benefit requirements, but have little data on consumers' experiences. *Commonwealth Fund.* http:// www.commonwealthfund.org/publications/blog/2015/oct/states-revisit-insurer-benefit -requirements-but-have-little-data-on-consumers-experiences. Published October 27, 2015. Accessed July 24, 2017.

75. Coverage of certain preventive services under the Affordable Care Act. 78 F.R. 127. 39870–39899 (July 2, 2013).

76. Pear R. Trump rule could deny birth control coverage to hundreds of thousands of women. *New York Times.* https://www.nytimes.com/2017/06/01/us/politics/birth-control-women -trump-health-care.html. Published June 1, 2017. Accessed July 24, 2017.

77. Guttmacher Institute. *Restricting insurance coverage of abortion.* https://www.guttmacher .org/state-policy/explore/restricting-insurance-coverage-abortion. Published July 1, 2017. Accessed July 24, 2017.

78. Guttmacher Institute. *Insurance coverage of contraception.* https://www.guttmacher.org /state-policy/explore/insurance-coverage-contraceptives. Published July 1, 2017. Accessed July 24, 2017.

79. Healthcare.gov. *How to pick a health insurance plan.* https://www.healthcare.gov/choose-a -plan/plans-categories/#catastrophic. Accessed August 7, 2017.

80. Kaiser Family Foundation. *Counties at risk for having no insurer on the marketplace (Exchange) in 2018.* http://www.kff.org/interactive/counties-at-risk-of-having-no-insurer -on-the-marketplace-exchange-in-2018/. Published June 20, 2017. Accessed July 31, 2017.

81. Office of Assistant Secretary for Planning and Evaluation. *2017 poverty guidelines for the 48 contiguous states and the District of Columbia.* https://aspe.hhs.gov/poverty-guidelines. Accessed July 24, 2017.

82. Kaiser Family Foundation. *Explaining health reform: questions about health insurance subsidies.* http://www.kff.org/healthreform/upload/7962-02.pdf. Published July 1, 2012. Accessed August 7, 2017.

83. Taylor A, Saenz A, Levine M. Supreme Court upholds Obamacare subsidies, President says ACA "Is Here to Stay." *ABC News.* http://abcnews.go.com/Politics/supreme-court-upholds -obama-health-care-subsidies/story?id=31931412. Accessed August 7, 2017.

84. Internal Revenue Service. Health Insurance Premium Tax Credit. 77 F.R. 30377. May 23, 2012.

85. *King v. Burwell,* No. 14–114.

86. Blumberg LJ, Holahan J, Buettgen M. *Why not just eliminate the employer mandate?* Washington, DC: Urban Institute. http://www.rwjf.org/content/dam/farm/reports/issue _briefs/2014/rwjf413248. Accessed August 7, 2017.

87. Goth G. ACA's effect on employment debated. *Society for Human Resource Management.* https://www.shrm.org/ResourcesAndTools/hr-topics/benefits/Pages/ACA-hiring-hours .aspx. Published Feb. 4, 2016. Accessed July 25, 2017.

88. National Conference of State Legislators. *States with effective rate review programs* http://www.ncsl .org/research/health/health-insurance-rate-approval-disapproval.aspx. Updated June 2016. Accessed July 25, 2017.

89. Interim Final Rule, Health Insurance Issuers Implementing Medical Loss Ratio Requirements Under the Patient Protection and Affordable Care Act, 75 F.R. 74864 (2010).

90. Healthcare.gov. *Grandfathered health insurance plans.* https://www.healthcare.gov/health -care-law-protections/grandfathered-plans/. Accessed July 25, 2017.

91. Families USA. *Grandfathered plans under the Patient Protection and Affordable Care Act.* http://familiesusa.org/product/grandfathered-plans-under-patient-protection-and -affordable-care-act. Accessed August 7, 2017.

92. Kaiser Family Foundation and Health Research and Educational Trust. *Employer health benefits: 2016.* http://www.kff.org/health-costs/report/2016-employer-health-benefits-survey/. Published September 14, 2016. Accessed July 25, 2017.

93. Health Reform Legislative Brief. *Self-insured plans under health reform.* http://www .ciswv.com/CIS/media/CISMedia/Documents/Self-Insured-Plans-Under-Health-Care -Reform-070312_1.pdf. Accessed August 7, 2017.

94. Department of Health and Human Services. *Prevention and Public Health Fund.* https://www .hhs.gov/open/prevention/index.html. Accessed August 8, 2017.

95. Trust for America's Health. *The prevention and public health fund: Preventing disease and reducing long-term health costs.* http://tfah.org/health-issues/wp-content/uploads/2017/05 /Fund-Backgrounder-May-17.pdf. Accessed July 25, 2017.

96. Abrams M, Nuzum R, Ryan J, Kiszla J, Guterman S. The Affordable Care Act's payment and systems delivery reforms: A progress report at five years. *The Commonwealth Fund.* http://www.commonwealthfund.org/publications/issue-briefs/2015/may/aca-payment-and -delivery-system-reforms-at-5-years. Published May 7, 2015. Accessed July 25, 2017.

97. *National Federation of Independent Business v. Sebelius,* 132 S.Ct. 2566 (2012).

98. *United States v. Lopez,* 514 U.S. 549 (1995) (possession of a gun near school is not an economic activity that has a substantial effect on interstate commerce); *United States v. Morrison,* 529 U.S. 598 (2000) (federal Violence Against Women Act of 1994 is unconstitutional violation of congressional Commerce Clause power).

99. Advisory Board. *Where states stand on Medicaid expansion.* https://www.advisory.com /daily-briefing/resources/primers/medicaidmap. Published May 19, 2017. Accessed July 25, 2017.

100. Medicaid, CHIP Payment and Access Commission. *Medicaid enrollment changes following the ACA.* https://www.macpac.gov/subtopic/medicaid-enrollment-changes-following-the-aca/. Accessed July 25, 2017.

101. Garfield R. The coverage gap: Uninsured poor adults in states that do not expand Medicaid. *Kaiser Family Foundation.* http://www.kff.org/uninsured/issue-brief/the-coverage-gap -uninsured-poor-adults-in-states-that-do-not-expand-medicaid/. Published October 19, 2016. Accessed July 25, 2017.

102. The American Health Care Act of 2017, H.R. 1628.

103. Fox L, Lee MJ, Mattingly P, Barrett T. Senate rejects proposals to repeal and replace Obamacare. *CNN.* http://www.cnn.com/2017/07/25/politics/senate-health-care-vote/index .html. Published July 26, 2017. Accessed July 26, 2017.

104. Lee MJ, Mattingly P. Health care debate: Senate rejects full Obamacare repeal without replacement. *CNN.* http://www.cnn.com/2017/07/26/politics/health-care-bill-wednesday /index.html. Published July 26, 2017. Accessed July 26, 2017.

105. Fox L. John McCain's maverick moment. *CNN.* http://www.cnn.com/2017/07/28/politics /john-mccain-maverick-health-care/index.html. Published July 26, 2017. Accessed July 31, 2017.

106. Congressional Budget Office. *Better Care Reconciliation Act of 2017—Cost Estimate.* https:// www.cbo.gov/system/files/115th-congress-2017-2018/costestimate/52849-hr1628senate.pdf. Published June 26, 2017. Accessed July 26, 2017.

107. Watkins E. Groups lining up in opposition to GOP health care plan. *CNN.* http://www.cnn .com/2017/03/08/politics/interest-groups-politicians-american-health-care-act/index.html. Published March 9, 2017. Accessed July 26, 2017.

108. Kaiser Family Foundation. *Health tracking poll July 2017: What's next for Republican ACA repeal and replacement plan efforts?* http://www.kff.org/health-reform/poll-finding/kaiser -health-tracking-poll-july-2017-whats-next-for-republican-aca-repeal-and-replacement -plan-efforts/. Published July 14, 2017. Accessed July 26, 2017.

109. Park M. Senator announces bipartisan hearing on Obamacare. *CNN.* http://www.cnn .com/2017/08/02/politics/senate-health-care-hearing-bipartisan/index.html. Published August 2, 2017. Accessed August 7, 2017.

110. Lee M. Bipartisan coalition looks to solve problem of individual market. *Modern Healthcare.* http://www.modernhealthcare.com/article/20170731/NEWS/170739986. Published July 31, 2017. Accessed August 7, 2017.

111. Kaiser Family Foundation. *The opioid epidemic and Medicaid's role in treatment: A look at changes over time.* http://www.kff.org/slideshow/the-opioid-epidemic-and-medicaids-role -in-treatment-a-look-at-changes-over-time/. Accessed July 26, 2017.

112. Sullivan P. Cornyn: Knowing health plan ahead of vote is "luxury we don't have." *The Hill.* http://thehill.com/policy/healthcare/342980-cornyn-knowing-health-plan-ahead-of-vote -is-luxury-we-dont-have. Published July 20, 2017. Accessed July 26, 2017.

113. Capehart J. Pelosi defends her infamous health care remark. *Washington Post.* https://www .washingtonpost.com/blogs/post-partisan/post/pelosi-defends-her-infamous-health-care -remark/2012/06/20/gJQAqch6qV_blog.html?utm_term=.6b4f042c53bb. Published June 12, 2012. Accessed July 26, 2017.

114. Tillett E. Trump on Senate's health care failure: "Let Obamacare fail." *CBS News.* http://www.cbsnews.com/news/trump-on-senates-health-care-failure-let-obamacare-fail/. Published July 18, 2017. Accessed July 26, 2017.

115. Jost T. Trump executive order on ACA: what it won't do, what it might do, and when. *Health Affairs Blog.* January 20, 2017. http://healthaffairs.org/blog/2017/01/20/trump-executive -order-on-aca-what-it-wont-do-what-it-might-do-and-when/. Accessed March 31, 2017.

116. Associated Press. *On Trump's order, IRS stops enforcing Obamacare fines.* http://www.nola.com /business/index.ssf/2017/02/on_trumps_order_irs_stops_enfo.html. Accessed April 3, 2017.

117. Jost T. Unpacking the Trump administration's market stabilization proposed rule. *Health Affairs Blog.* February 16, 2017. http://healthaffairs.org/blog/2017/02/16/unpacking-the -trump-administrations-market-stabilization-proposed-rule/. Accessed April 4, 2017.

118. Newkirk VR. Obamacare isn't out of the woods yet. *The Atlantic.* https://www.theatlantic.com /politics/archive/2017/03/the-aca-isnt-out-of-the-woods-yet/520830/. Accessed April 3, 2017.

119. Bagely N, McIntyre A. Executive actions Trump could take to change the ACA. *The Incidental Economist.* http://theincidentaleconomist.com/wordpress/executive-actions-trump-could-take -to-change-the-aca/. Accessed April 3, 2017.

120. Pear B, Abelson R. Health subsidies for low-earners will continue through 2017, G.O.P. says. *The New York Times.* March 30, 2017. https://www.nytimes.com/2017/03/30/us/politics /health-insurance-republicans.html. Accessed March 31, 2017.

121. Mangan D. California will allow insurers to file two sets of rates: One for 'Trumpcare,' other for 'Obamacare.' *CNBC.* http://www.cnbc.com/2017/04/28/california-will-allow-health -insurers-to-file-two-sets-of-rates-one-for-trumpcare-other-for-obamacare.html. Published April 28, 2017. Accessed July 26, 2017.

122. Adamczyk A. Here's how much Obamacare premiums will increase in 2018. *Money.* http://time.com/money/4826591/aca-premiums-cost-2018/. Published June 22, 2017. Accessed July 26, 2017.

123. Livingston S. Health insurers' proposed 2018 rate hikes are early warning signs. *Modern Healthcare.* http://www.modernhealthcare.com/article/20170510/NEWS/170519999/. Published May 10, 2017. Accessed July 26, 2017.

124. Luhby T. Repeal is dead (for now). But will Obamacare survive? *CNN Money.* http://money. cnn.com/2017/07/29/news/economy/obamacare-repeal/index.html. Published July 29, 2017. Accessed July 31, 2017.

125. Fise P. Cost sharing reduction subsidies: What happens if they aren't paid? *Bipartisan Policy Center.* https://bipartisanpolicy.org/blog/cost-sharing-reduction-subsidies-what-happens-if -they-arent-paid/. Published June 8, 2017. Accessed July 26, 2017.

126. Tajlili B. Premiums to rise in 2018 for Affordable Care Act plans. *Blue Cross Blue Shield of North Carolina.* http://blog.bcbsnc.com/2017/05/premiums-rise-2018-affordable-care-act -plans/. Published May 25, 2017. Accessed July 31, 2017.

127. Levy G. Last 'bare' county in US to have Obamacare coverage in 2018. *US News and World Report.* https://www.usnews.com/news/national-news/articles/2017-08-24/last-bare-county-in -us-to-have-obamacare-coverage-in-2018. Published August 24, 2017. Accessed August 30, 2017.

128. Cox C, Levitt L. Individual insurance market performance in early 2017. *Kaiser Family Foundation.* http://www.kff.org/health-reform/issue-brief/individual-insurance-market -performance-in-early-2017/. Published July 10, 2017. Accessed July 31, 2017.

129. McKinsey Center for Health System Reform. Exchanges three years in: Market variations and factors affecting performance. http://healthcare.mckinsey.com/sites/default/files /Intel%20Brief%20-%20Individual%20Market%20Performance%20and%20Outlook%20 %28public%29_vF.pdf. Published May 13, 2016. Accessed July 31, 2017.

130. Zeitlin J. Are the ACA exchanges really in a death spiral? We asked the experts. *Advisory Board.* https://www.advisory.com/daily-briefing/2017/02/16/death-exchange-market. Published February 16, 2017. Accessed July 31, 2017.